GOLF Rx

Also by Vijay Vad, M.D.

ARTHRITIS RX

BACK RX

GOLF Rx

A FIFTEEN-MINUTE-A-DAY CORE PROGRAM
FOR MORE YARDS AND LESS PAIN

Vijay Vad, M.D.,
with DAVE ALLEN

GOTHAM
BOOKS

GOTHAM BOOKS
Published by Penguin Group (USA) Inc.
375 Hudson Street, New York, New York 10014, U.S.A.

Penguin Group (Canada), 90 Eglinton Avenue East, Suite 700, Toronto, Ontario, Canada M4P 2Y3 (a division of Pearson Penguin Canada Inc.); Penguin Books Ltd, 80 Strand, London WC2R 0RL, England; Penguin Ireland, 25 St Stephen's Green, Dublin 2, Ireland (a division of Penguin Books Ltd); Penguin Group (Australia), 250 Camberwell Road, Camberwell, Victoria 3124, Australia (a division of Pearson Australia Group Pty Ltd); Penguin Books India Pvt Ltd, 11 Community Centre, Panchsheel Park, New Delhi – 110 017, India; Penguin Group (NZ), 67 Apollo Drive, Rosedale, North Shore 0632, New Zealand (a division of Pearson New Zealand Ltd); Penguin Books (South Africa) (Pty) Ltd, 24 Sturdee Avenue, Rosebank, Johannesburg 2196, South Africa

Penguin Books Ltd, Registered Offices: 80 Strand, London WC2R 0RL, England

Published by Gotham Books, a member of Penguin Group (USA) Inc.

Previously published as a Gotham Books hardcover edition

First trade paperback printing, March 2008

10 9 8 7 6 5 4 3 2

Gotham Books and the skyscraper logo are trademarks of Penguin Group (USA) Inc.

THE LIBRARY OF CONGRESS HAS CATALOGED THE HARDCOVER EDITION AS FOLLOWS:

Vad, Vijay.
    Golf Rx : a 15-minute-a-day core program for more yards and less pain / Vijay Vad, with Dave Allen.
        p. cm.
    ISBN: 978-1-592-40266-3 (hardcover)   ISBN: 978-1-592-40340-0 (paperback)
    1. Golfers—Health and hygiene.   2. Golf injuries—Prevention.   3. Golf—Physiological aspects.
    I. Allen, Dave, 1968–   II. Title.
    RC1220.G64V33   2007
    617.1'027—dc22   2006027207

Printed in the United States of America
Set in Electra

To my beautiful daughter Amoli.
May she appreciate good sportsmanship
and strive to leave the world a better place
than how she found it.

CONTENTS

INTRODUCTION
THE *GOLF Rx* WAY TO A BETTER SWING

A few summers ago, I received an emergency phone call from a fifty-two-year-old patient of mine who had collapsed on the 17th green at Shinnecock Hills Golf Club (site of the 2004 U.S. Open) on Long Island. He was about to putt for a birdie when he reached down to pick up his marker and suddenly crumpled to the ground in a heap, pain radiating through his buttocks and down his right leg.

After being taken by ambulance to the local emergency room, he was transported back to the Hospital for Special Surgery in New York, where I treated him for a bulging disk in his lower back. The disk was pressing up against his sciatic nerve, causing tremendous pain and immobility. After giving him an epidural injection at the spot where the nerve and protruding disk met, he was standing again. That was the good news. The bad news: It would be about two months before he'd be attempting another birdie putt.

In this particular instance, it was early in the season, the golfer had only a round or two under his belt, and his body was in no condition to handle the rigors associated with playing eighteen holes of golf. He had been golf deconditioned after several months away from the game, and he was hurrying back too soon without getting his body in golf shape.

I've seen this type of injury countless times in my ten years as a physician at the Hospital for Special Surgery, a world-renowned sports medicine institution that provides services for the ATP men's professional tennis circuit, the U.S. swimming and rowing teams, the New York Mets baseball team, the New York Knicks basketball team, and the New York Giants football team, among others. During that time, I've treated more than 3,000 golfers, half of them with back-related injuries. It is the most common sports injury I see among fifty- and sixty-year-old men. In fact, it is estimated that half of all recreational golfers and one-third of all professional golfers suffer from some form of lower-back pain.

In my role as a consulting physician for the PGA Tour, the tour asked me in 2001 to conduct a study on the causes of lower-back pain in professional golfers. It was a parallel study to the one I conducted on the ATP tennis tour in 1999–2000. Up until this time, it was widely believed that the violent, twisting nature of the golf swing and the tremendous forces imparted on the spine were the cause of lower-back problems. But our research showed that the back was only partially to blame.

We tested forty-two PGA Tour professionals at the 2001 Buick Classic (now referred to as the Barclays Classic, for which I serve as the medical director) in Westchester County, New York, and found that those who suffered from lower-back pain had substantially less flexibility in their lead hip—the left hip for right-handed golfers—versus their trailing hip. In those players who didn't suffer from lower-back pain, the lead-hip discrepancy wasn't as significant.

This made a whole lot of sense because in the golf swing, rapid deceleration takes place the moment you contact the ball. In less than a second, your swing goes from eighty- to ninety-plus miles per hour to a complete stop. Just try asking your car to do that without burning the rubber on your tires down to the pavement! If there's little range of motion in your lead hip, your body is not going to be able to withstand these deceleration forces very well, and your back will become the primary shock absorber. These deceleration forces have to be absorbed by your whole body, and if one part of that system (your hips) is not doing its job, it's going to move on to the next part of the system, which is your lower back, and so on. The key is that you don't want so many forces getting to your back so soon; you want them to dissipate before they get there.

It was from this research published in the prestigious *American Journal of Sports Medicine* that *Golf Rx* was born, which makes it the first golf-fitness book on the market today based on a clinical study of PGA Tour professionals. *Golf Rx* contains three step-by-step exercise series and more than eighty core-specific exercises designed to increase the range of motion in your lead hip, as well as improve your overall flexibility, strength, and endurance so that you can enjoy the game pain-free for the duration of the season—and longer.

However, *Golf Rx* is more than a book about injury prevention; it seeks to improve your performance on the course as well. By progressing through the golf-specific exercise programs, you will hit the ball farther and straighter than ever before. Your swing mechanics will improve, and so will your consistency of play and your ball-striking. In this aspect, *Golf Rx* is different from my first two books, *Back Rx* and *Arthritis Rx*. It is not only a book about treating pain and preventing future injuries, it's about improving your level of play so you can break 90 or 80 for the first time in your life, regardless of your age.

The thing I most admire about golf is that it's a lifetime recreational activity, one you can enjoy well into your later years if you stay healthy. In that sense, there's no other sport like it. And, thanks to today's technology—lighter metals and shafts, gorilla-size clubheads, and balls that fly to the moon—golfers are constantly offered new ways to improve, and fast. *Golf Rx* will also help you to do that.

The golf-specific exercises in Series A, B, and C will help you achieve both your fitness and performance goals, no matter what your skill or interest level. Whether you're a beginning golfer just looking to increase your flexibility and range of motion (Series A), an intermediate golfer looking to add ten to twenty more yards to your drives (Series B), or an advanced golfer seeking to improve your endurance and maximize performance (Series C), *Golf Rx* is for you. The best part is that you can perform these exercises at home, in front of your television, or in your hotel room. You don't have to belong to a gym, and you don't need to lift any heavy weights. Some shorts, a T-shirt, and the occasional golf club is all you need.

In addition to the routines in Series A, B, and C, *Golf Rx* also contains exercises to help you warm up (Chapter Five) and cool down (Chapter Seven) before and after you play, so that you don't return to the course the next day as stiff as your 5-iron. There are stretches for every hole on the golf course (Chapter Six), just in case you find yourself waiting to tee off or you feel a need for a mental time-out. There are full chapters devoted to the mental side of the game (Chapter Nine) and to nutrition (Chapter Ten), and for you John Daly wannabes, there are fourteen power exercises in Chapter Four designed to stretch out your drives so you can blow it by your buddies off the tee.

The perfect preseason conditioning program, *Golf Rx* enables you to safely and efficiently generate power. Combine that with good swing mechanics, and you will play your best golf ever—and pain-free, too.

PART ONE

PERFORMANCE
ENHANCEMENT

CHAPTER ONE

PROPER BODY MECHANICS FOR A GOOD GOLF SWING

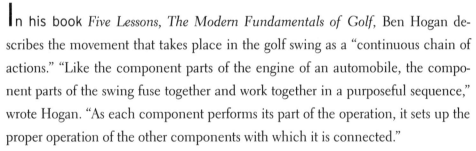

In his book *Five Lessons, The Modern Fundamentals of Golf,* Ben Hogan describes the movement that takes place in the golf swing as a "continuous chain of actions." "Like the component parts of the engine of an automobile, the component parts of the swing fuse together and work together in a purposeful sequence," wrote Hogan. "As each component performs its part of the operation, it sets up the proper operation of the other components with which it is connected."

Proper sequencing is the key to making a timely, powerful golf swing. For example, in the forward swing the first body part to move is your legs, followed by your hips, shoulders, and, finally, your arms and hands. Your hands transfer the power you've generated up to that point to the club. If that sequence is broken (for example, if your hands start down first), or there's a glitch in the kinematic chain, your ability to hit the ball solidly is greatly diminished. And there is very little room for error: Miss the center of the clubface by as little as a quarter of an inch, or even less, and you can find yourself in the trees with the chipmunks instead of in the fairway.

Get the sequencing correct, and you strongly enhance your chances of hitting the center of the clubface and finding the heart of the fairway.

The ultimate goal is to perform the correct movements automatically without having to think so much, to repeat your swing under pressure as though it were on autopilot.

The following swing sequence of Vijay Singh, shot in 2004 at the Mercedes Championships in Hawaii, will help give you a better understanding of the proper movements, or biomechanics, required of your body during the swing. It's Vijay at his very best—he shot to number one in the Official World Golf Ranking in '04 and also captured PGA Tour Player of the Year honors with nine victories and more than $10 million in earnings.

This chapter will analyze in detail eight key positions in Vijay's swing—from address to the finish. You will learn the proper sequencing of movement that will allow you to make a full backswing. You will also learn why it's important to keep the clubhead lagging behind your hands well into the downswing, and what it means to clear your hips.

Of course, not everyone is built like Vijay, nor do they have the time to spend four to five hours a day hitting balls on the practice range, as he's known to do. But with a better understanding of the fundamental movements of a tour player's swing, you'll gain an appreciation for the golf-specific exercises you'll see later in this book, and why they're being prescribed for you.

ADDRESS: THE FOUNDATION

Your address position, or how you stand to the ball, lays the groundwork for your swing. It impacts your body's movement, the path the clubhead takes during the swing, your balance, the clubhead speed, and the point at which the clubface makes contact with the ball. In other words, it's the most important position in golf. "Set up correctly," wrote Jack Nicklaus in *Golf My Way*, and "there's a good chance

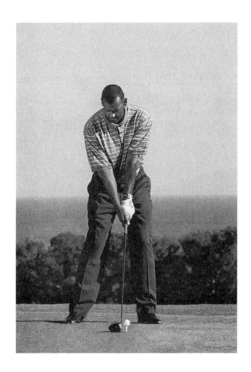 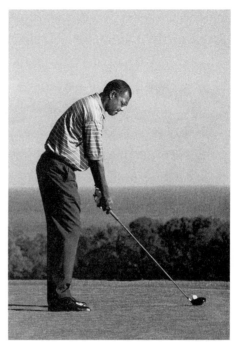

you'll hit a reasonable shot, even if you make a mediocre swing. Set up incorrectly, and you'll hit a lousy shot even if you make the greatest swing in the world."

The angles created by your body at address form the foundation of a good setup. In the photo above (left), you'll see that Vijay's spine angles to the right, away from the target. This lowers his right shoulder, which mirrors the position of his right hand on the club—below his left. More importantly, it presets his upper body behind the ball, so that he has an easier time loading his weight onto his right side and turning his shoulders. It also presets his body in the correct impact position, with his head and upper body behind the ball, so that he can transfer maximum force to the ball.

Vijay tilts forward from his hips—about 30 to 35 degrees—so that his chest points toward the ground. This directly impacts the path, or plane, the club will take during the swing. Hogan referred to this plane as a tilted pane of glass running from the ball through the top of your shoulders. It is also frequently defined as the angle your shaft makes when soled on the ground at address. Your club is considered to be on-plane when your shaft travels parallel to this tilted line during the swing. The more on-plane your swing is, the flatter your angle of approach is into the ball and the more clubhead speed and power you're able to generate.

If you stand too erect at address, your shoulders will swing on a more horizontal plane and there will be little downward movement to the club. You'll have to significantly alter your posture during the downswing to get down to the ball. Bend over too much at address, and your plane will be more vertical—almost straight up and down. Consequently, you'll have a hard time turning your shoulders and delivering the club from the inside with any speed or accuracy.

Provided Vijay maintains his forward tilt, he should be able to rotate his shoulders and pelvis back and through with maximum speed and efficiency, without having to make any compensations to his swing. His shoulders will remain on-plane, helping to deliver the clubhead from the proper inside path for a solid hit on the ball.

Vijay's weight is centered over both feet, just forward of his arches, which creates good balance and the desired swing path. Put too much weight on your toes and you'll pick the club up too steeply; too much toward your heels and you'll swing the club too far to the inside. His stance width, which is measured by the distance between his heels, is widest with his driver and narrowest with his wedges, or shortest clubs. A wider stance helps support a longer swing and encourages a bigger swing arc and more clubhead speed. A narrow stance restricts the amount of shoulder turn you can generate in the backswing but increases your body rotation through impact.

TAKEAWAY: SMOOTH FROM THE START

Vijay starts the club back with the big muscles of his chest and shoulders; his hips are the last to move. In fact, there's little movement to his hips during the first few feet of his backswing. His lower body remains very quiet, as though it were cast in

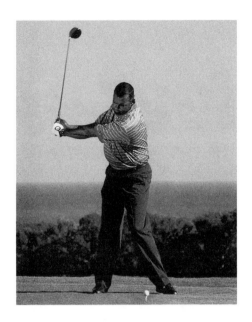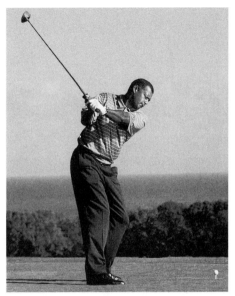

cement. Vijay's left arm remains snug against his chest as he turns back, which helps keep the clubhead outside of his hands and on-plane. This is the primary function of the takeaway—to get the club started back on the proper plane, with good rhythm and tempo. Vijay also gets great extension with his arms, which creates a bigger, wider swing arc and more power.

HALFWAY BACK: CREATING LEVERAGE

By the time his arms are parallel to the ground, Vijay's wrists are fully hinged, creating a 90-degree angle between the shaft and his left forearm (*above, left*). This is leverage that he will use later in his swing to unleash his explosive power. Vijay's hands remain in front of his chest, an indication that everything is moving back together in the proper sequence, and the butt end of the club points at the ball (*above, right*), again signifying that the club is on-plane.

What is most interesting about Vijay's swing here is his left-knee position. Singh fully releases his knee behind the ball, which, as you will see in the next set of

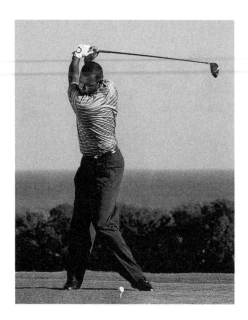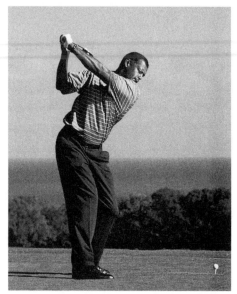

photographs (*above*), allows him to make an enormous hip turn and an even greater shoulder turn as he reaches the top of his backswing.

TOP OF BACKSWING: THE WINDUP

This is one backswing every amateur should emulate, says CBS television commentator and renowned instructor Peter Kostis, because it doesn't require Gumby-like flexibility. Vijay's left heel comes off the ground, which allows him to rotate his hips and shoulders so far back. It is the classic "turn inside the barrel" image made famous by Percy Boomer: Vijay's right hip pivots straight back, without bumping into the side of an imaginary waist-high barrel, while his shoulders rotate perpendicular to his spine. His left shoulder turns very deeply, directly over his right knee, setting the stage for a very powerful unwinding of his hips and shoulders on the downswing.

From a down-the-line view, you'll notice that Vijay maintains the same forward tilt he established at address (*above, right*). The clubface is parallel to his

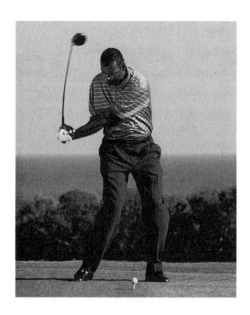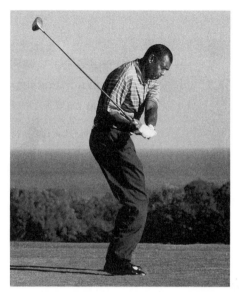

left forearm, which means it's square and in perfect position to start the downswing.

FIRST MOVE DOWN: THE HIPS UNWIND

Unlike the backswing, the lower body initiates the downswing; the upper body is the last to unwind. The hips start to clear, or open—rotating back to the left of the body—followed by the shoulders. As the hips unwind, they free up space for the arms to swing down freely from the inside. Vijay's right foot and knee roll inward, toward the target, while his left foot remains planted on the ground. This way, his lower body stays more underneath him, so that he can release and fire his right side through. Again, it's the classic "turn inside the barrel" swing, as his left hip unwinds without sliding too far past the ball to bump the side of the barrel. Vijay's wrists remain fully hinged and the clubhead lags well behind his hands (*above, left*), which stores tremendous leverage (the angle between his left forearm and the shaft is more than 100 degrees!) and power that he will unload at impact.

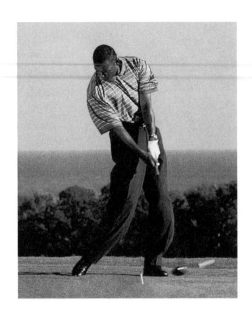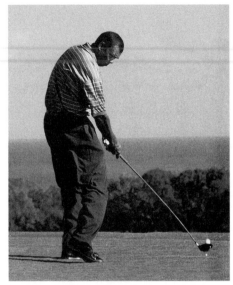

IMPACT: STRAIGHTEN THE ANGLE

The angle between Vijay's left forearm and the shaft in the previous set of photos is now a straight line, extending upward from the clubhead through his left shoulder. It is this straightening out of the angle through impact that gives Vijay the additional burst of clubhead speed he needs to routinely drive the ball 300 yards (Singh averaged 301.1 yards per drive on the PGA Tour in 2005). It's similar to snapping a whip: The longer you can keep the clubhead lagging behind your hands in the downswing, the more energy you'll transfer to the ball at impact. WARNING: As soon as the clubhead passes the hands, the club loses speed.

From behind, you can see almost all of Vijay's backside, which shows you how completely rotated he is. His hips have cleared about 45 degrees while his shoulders are just starting to open, or catch up (*above, right*). This is the result of good sequencing in the downswing: Your hips should unwind first, then your shoulders. Keep your shoulders turned back—closed, or pointing right of the target—as you start to rotate your hips back toward the target. The more separation you get between your hips and shoulders as you change direction, the faster you'll be able to unwind your body and swing the club.

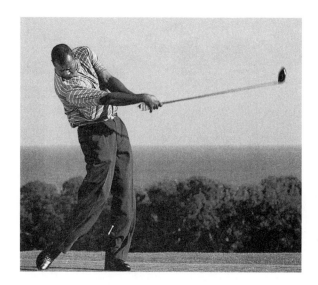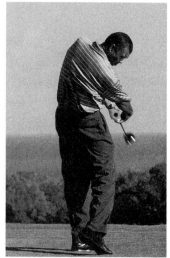

HALFWAY THROUGH: EXTEND THE ARMS

Vijay's left leg forms a firm post, which enables him to rotate his upper body around to the left and into the finish. Both arms are extended toward the target, and his forearms appear to be almost touching (*above, left*), a sign of a good release—the right forearm rotating over the left and squaring the clubface. He maintains his shoulder tilt (indicated by stripes on his shirt) well into the follow-through, so that the shaft is on the same plane it was at address and at impact. The hips are still turning to the left and his upper body is moving in the same direction, pulling the club around to his left.

FINISH: THE END RESULT

The finish is a by-product of everything that happens before it. If you have good balance, you should be able to hold your finish position for a count of five, which Vijay can do very easily. Most of his weight has settled on his left foot, whereas only his big toe touches the ground on his right foot. His thighs face forward—actually, left of the target—and appear to be glued together, an indication that Vijay has rotated

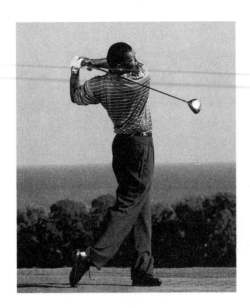 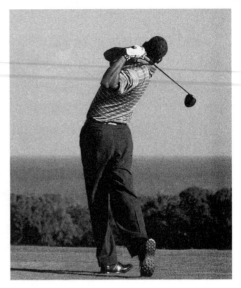

his lower body all the way through. From straight on, you can see his right shoulder is closer to the target than his left. This means he's done a good job of rotating his upper body through as well. His forward tilt is the same as it was at address, something that wouldn't be possible without proper sequencing, good balance, and a strong, flexible core, all of which Vijay possesses.

SUMMARY POINTS

Here's a quick overview of the eight key positions in the golf swing, and what you should try to accomplish with each one. Remember: No two golf swings are exactly the same, and some are quite unusual, albeit very effective. PGA Tour veteran Jim Furyk's swing has been likened to an "octopus falling out of a tree"—in the words of CBS commentator David Feherty—but it hasn't stopped him from winning a U.S. Open and many more PGA Tour events. The most important thing is to get your swing to repeat and work for you. The following pointers will help:

- *Address:* Make sure to angle your spine away from the target, which presets your upper body behind the ball. Tilt your spine more for a driver and less for a wedge.
- *Takeaway:* Start the club back with the larger muscles of your body, and keep your lower body quiet, as though it's in cement.
- *Halfway Back:* Hinge your wrists so that your left forearm and the clubshaft form a 90-degree angle.
- *Top of Backswing:* Turn your left shoulder over your right knee without losing your posture (or forward tilt) from address. If you're not very flexible, allow your left heel to come slightly off the ground with the longer clubs.
- *First Move Down:* Start the downswing from the ground up, keeping your shoulders turned back as long as you can while unwinding your lower body.
- *Impact:* Allow the clubhead to accelerate gradually so it's moving at its maximum speed when it reaches the ball. Keep the clubhead lagging behind your hands for as long as you can, which creates an extra burst of speed through the hitting zone.
- *Halfway Through:* Extend your arms toward the target while swinging the club around to the left of your body.
- *Finish:* Rotate your upper body through so that your right shoulder points toward the target at the completion of your swing. Almost all of your weight should rest on your left foot.

CHAPTER TWO

CORE STABILITY: THE ENGINE THAT DRIVES AND *BRAKES* YOUR SWING

A Boeing 747 jet will reach cruising speeds of 500-plus miles per hour. The average golfer, on the other hand, will top out at about 90 miles per hour of clubhead speed. The difference is that the jumbo jet will start its descent and initial slowdown phase about twenty to thirty minutes before landing; the average golfer will have less than a second to come to a complete stop. There is no gradual deceleration; your body has to brake itself in about the time it takes you to unbuckle your seat belt.

The primary job of applying the brakes in this rapid deceleration phase belongs to the core, a collection of muscles and tendons located between your thighs and chest, or where your upper and lower body meet. The core works to stabilize and absorb these deceleration forces to your spine so that you don't incur an injury. The more fatigued your core becomes, the more likely you are to sustain a serious injury.

"Muscles are not only responsible for moving you, they're responsible for stopping you," says Paul Schueren, a physical therapist with the PGA Tour. "As much as the core is an accelerator, it's also a decelerator."

For the most part, the core muscles in the front of your body are your accelerators, or thrusters, to use an airplane analogy again. They transmit power to your shoulders and upper torso, which in turn transfer energy to your arms and fingers and, finally, the golf club. These accelerators include your hip flexors, quadriceps, glutes, and abdominals. Your posterior muscles are the all-important decelerators, or reverse thrusters. These include your primary back muscles, or paraspinals, hamstrings, and internal hip rotators.

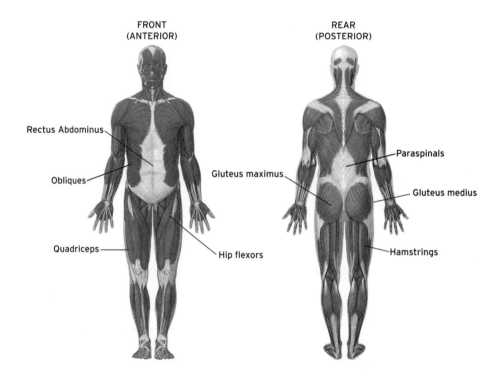

This is why it's essential not to ignore your backside when conditioning your body, even if it isn't seen as important as your chest and abs—nor viewed as often. A lot of people confuse the core with the abdominal muscles. They think that if they do sit-ups and crunches all day long, they'll have a strong, well-functioning core.

But it takes much more than a six-pack of abs to hit a golf ball 300 yards. Your abdominal muscles compose just a small part of your core, and you need your entire core to do its job to hit the cover off of the ball. And do it safely. When you swing a club, your glutes, hip flexors, paraspinals, quadriceps, and hamstrings are all firing, just as your abs are. So, while a chiseled stomach is great to show off at the beach, it isn't going to help you bring the club to a stop safely if the rest of your core is weak or not conditioned properly.

ACCELERATORS AND DECELERATORS

Glutes: The Workhorse Muscles

Any discussion of the golf-specific core muscles has to start with your glutes, or buttocks, because they are not only major accelerators, they also work equally hard in the deceleration phase of the swing. There are three muscles that make up your

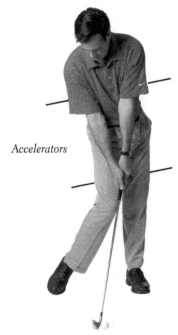

Accelerators

Your core is your primary power source and braking mechanism.

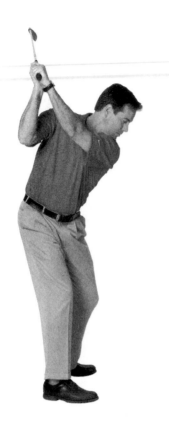

glutes: the gluteus maximus, gluteus medius, and gluteus minimus. The gluteus maximus is the true gladiator of the three, because it is the strongest muscle in the human body. It's also the largest muscle in the core, and as such is a very powerful rotator and producer of speed. It not only provides a cushion for you to sit on, it also helps rotate your hips from side to side, and acts as a strong stabilizer for your trunk and pelvis.

The gluteus medius lies on the outside of your hip, directly above the gluteus maximus. It assists in moving your hips laterally, away from your body's midline (an example would be when you shift your weight forward on the downswing), and also helps you bend from the hips. The gluteus minimus is the innermost of the three gluteal muscles, and also assists in rotating your hips internally, toward your midline (your right hip rotates internally during the backswing, as in the picture above), and externally.

Abdominals: Your Six-pack and Much More

As I stated earlier, the core is composed of more than just the abdominals, as many people are led to believe. But the abs still play a prominent role in the golf swing, especially the lower abs, which help to stabilize your trunk as well as rotate and bend your torso.

There are three groups of abdominal muscles. The largest and most visually appealing of these, and the one that sells millions of magazines, is the rectus abdominus, which extends from the top of the pelvis (pubic bone) to your sternum. The primary function of this muscle, besides making you look good, is to flex the trunk and help stabilize your spine. Thus, it works mostly as a decelerator.

The deepest and perhaps most undertrained of the abdominal muscles is the transverse abdominus, which runs across the sides of your body from your stomach to your back. Another big trunk stabilizer and decelerator, this muscle can be worked simply by drawing your belly button in toward your spine.

The accelerators are the obliques, which flank your rectus abdominus on both sides of your abdomen. The outermost abdominals are the external obliques, which run diagonally from front to back, forming a "V." They help you bend to the side, and also assist in rotating your trunk. The internal obliques lie underneath the external obliques, just inside your hips, and form an inverted "V." Like the external obliques, they are known as mobilizers, or muscles that move bone, and they help twist your torso from side to side.

ACCELERATORS

Hip Flexors: Overcoming the Desk-Job Syndrome

The primary accelerators in the swing are the hip flexors, or iliopsoas. Located deep in your thighs, these muscles attach to your femur and extend up into your lower abdominals, crossing the front of the hip joint. In fact, they are often confused with the lower abs because they are so deep in the core.

The hip flexors have two golf-specific functions: 1) They allow you to bend forward from the hip joints, drawing you closer to the ball, and 2) they work as external rotators to help move your trunk. This is why they're such big accelerators. However, the hip flexors are very prone to fatigue and tightness, because most of the time they sit in a prolonged, shortened state. I refer to this as the "desk-job syndrome." So many golfers live a sedentary lifestyle outside of the course, and this only works against the hip flexors. If they are not stretched regularly, they lose their elasticity, severely limiting your ability to get into extension and rotate your trunk effectively.

Quadriceps: Pillars of Strength

The primary function of this large muscle group at the front of your thigh is to extend the legs. In the golf swing, however, the quads play a vital role in maintaining your posture, or forward spine tilt. They form two strong pillars, creating a stable platform for you to swing around. If the quads are weak, it's very difficult to keep your knees flexed and maintain the correct distance from the ball. The longer you're able to maintain your posture, the more consistent your contact point will be, and the faster you'll be able to swing.

Hip External Rotators

There is a six-pack of smaller muscles located deep in your buttocks known as the hip external rotators. Their primary function, as their name suggests, is to rotate your hips and legs outward, both in the backswing and forward swing. These muscles include the quadratus femoris, obturators internus and externus, gemelli superior and inferior, and piriformis. The most well-known of these external rotators is the piriformis, which is located at the back of the hip joint. Besides being an important accelerator, the piriformis also helps to stabilize the pelvis, so you can sustain your posture and keep your lower body more underneath you throughout the swing. If this muscle is allowed to get too tight, it can irritate the sciatic nerve directly underneath it, causing pain or numbness in your buttocks and legs—also known as piriformis syndrome.

DECELERATORS

Paraspinals: The Spine's Primary Line of Defense

There's no sense having a car that goes 180 miles per hour if you don't have a set of high-performance brakes. In the golf swing, the paraspinals are those high-performance brakes. Located on both sides of your spinal column, these stabilizers work with your glutes to slow down your torso once the ball is hit. This way, your lower back doesn't take the full brunt of the twister created by so much clubhead speed. If these muscles are unable to help absorb the rapid deceleration forces that take place in the swing, you won't be playing golf much longer.

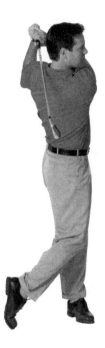

Hamstrings: Not to Be Ignored

It's not uncommon to see athletes with very well-defined quadriceps and weak, underdeveloped hamstrings, the large muscles at the back of your thigh. The explanation for this is simple: People like to look good up front. But this inequality that often exists between the two can lead to a major injury if you continue to ignore your hamstrings. The tighter these muscles are, the harder it is to bend forward from your hips and get down to the ball, and the more difficult it is to maintain your posture throughout the swing.

Besides extending the hips, the hamstrings also assist in rotating your pelvis. This is very important in the deceleration phase of the swing, because it allows you to fully release your right side through, reducing the amount of torque, or bending, on your lower back.

Hip Internal Rotators: The Back Brakes

The internal rotators of the hip, which include the gluteus medius, gluteus minimus, and tensor fascia latae, play an extremely important role in slowing your body down during the swing. As soon as you hit the ball, these brakes are turned on, pulling your hips in toward your body just as they start to move farther away from

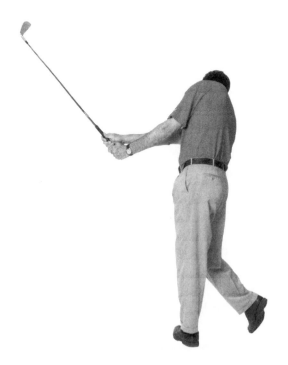

Your glutes work as decelerators.

THE CORE ESSENTIALS

Much like a baseball pitcher relies on his arm, or a soccer player on his legs, the golfer needs a well-conditioned core to play golf. It is the engine that makes peak golf performance possible, and it protects the vital muscular and skeletal structures needed to make a swing against injury. The more conditioned your core is, the more power and control you'll have over your swing, and the less likely you will be to sustain an injury. The core muscles—which include the glutes, abdominals, hip flexors, and hamstrings, among others—not only produce bursts of power, but also serve as shock absorbers and brakes to slow the body down and avoid injuries.

This chapter, combined with our PGA Tour research, is the foundation upon which the *Golf Rx* program is built. You will need to refer back to this chapter as you go through each series, as well as for many of the exercises in this book. By learning about the golf-specific core muscles and each of their vital functions, you will have a better understanding of your own swing and how to improve it.

the center line of your body. Essentially, they are pulling your hips ashore instead of letting them drift out too far, which puts tremendous strain on the lower back. In the backswing, it's the right hip that rotates internally while the left hip works externally, and in the downswing, the roles are reversed: The left hip has the primary responsibility of slowing your body down.

CHAPTER THREE

THE EFFECT OF AGING AND LIFESTYLE ON YOUR POSTURE

Imagine a stick of your favorite chewing gum. When you first put it in your mouth, the gum is supple and juicy, and it retains its size. You can blow big bubbles that practically cover your face. But after about thirty minutes of constant chewing, the gum is smaller and less flexible, and the bubbles you force out are at best the size of a golf ball.

Your body's muscular system is much like a piece of chewing gum. The older you get, the shorter and more rigid your muscles become. They begin to lose their elasticity and their ability to stretch, which means they cannot generate as much clubhead speed and power. Perhaps more importantly, they can't absorb forces like they used to, which makes you more susceptible to injury.

This process of muscle decline begins to pick up speed after the age of forty. About this time, you start to lose approximately 1 percent of muscle mass per year. In men, this is caused by a steady decline in testosterone, the hormone responsible for increasing the size of your muscle cells as you work out. In women, it's created by a loss of testosterone and estrogen, the primary female sex hormone.

You're going to lose muscle mass no matter what you do—it's a natural effect of aging—but you can minimize the loss by following exercise programs such as *Golf Rx*, working out on a regular basis (with a major emphasis on resistance training), and taking in the right foods and nutrients. What you can't do is drink lots of beer and exercise one or two days per week like you did as an undergrad and still expect to perform at a high level. That won't cut it anymore, and it certainly won't help your golf game.

The other obstacle confronting you at forty is that your tissues begin to lose water—about 1 percent per year. Your whole musculoskeletal shock-absorbing system—joints, muscles, tendons, ligaments, disks—becomes less hydrated and, therefore, less flexible and powerful. It begins to show signs of wear and tear, creating a degenerative cascade that can lead to serious back problems and injuries. The tendons your muscles attach to begin to lose their elasticity, which can lead to ruptures of the Achilles, patella, and other primary weight-bearing tendons. Instead of being full and moist, the disks in your back start to dry up and shrink. As a result, the facet joints in your lower back start to take on more stress.

Unfortunately, you cannot rehydrate these tissues by drinking more water, but you can slow down the degenerative cascade significantly by keeping your weight down, following a proper diet that includes fruits and vegetables, drinking plenty of water, and performing the exercises in *Golf Rx*. Just because you're getting older doesn't mean that you don't have some great golf left in you. That's hardly the case. Some professional golfers just start to hit their prime after turning forty. Vijay Singh enjoyed his best season ever at the age of forty-one in 2004, winning nine times and collecting more than $10 million in earnings on the PGA Tour. He also claimed the number-one ranking in the world from Tiger Woods in '04. Mark O'Meara was forty-one in 1998 when he captured the only two major championships of his career—the Masters and the British Open. And what about Hale Irwin? Since joining the Champions Tour in 1995, the sixty-year-old has collected more than $22.5 million (through 2005).

Irwin, a former football player at the University of Colorado, still works out regularly. And Vijay is probably in the best shape of his career—he has to be to log the countless hours he spends day after day on the practice range.

These players didn't let the natural aging process hinder them from obtaining their goals, and neither should you. With the help of *Golf Rx*, you can improve your golf performance, no matter what your age. *Golf Rx* can't help you become Vin Diesel or the Rock, but it can help you maintain good posture, flexibility, and strength, helping you to play good golf at any age.

POSTURE PITFALLS

As you get older, it becomes increasingly more difficult to maintain good posture for one golf swing, let alone an entire round of golf. The loss of water and elasticity in your muscles, tendons, and ligaments causes your body to shrink, drawing your center of gravity closer to the ball. Your body has a natural tendency to bend more,

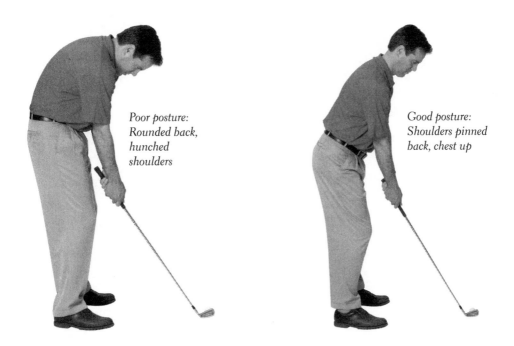

Poor posture: Rounded back, hunched shoulders

Good posture: Shoulders pinned back, chest up

or go into a state of flexion, which creates several swing problems. For one, the more bent or hunched over the ball you are, the harder it is to extend your arms through impact. To compensate, you will more than likely raise up out of your posture, or spine angle, to create enough distance between you and the ball so your arms can get into extension. Unfortunately, this leads to a lot of mishits and inconsistent results.

Also, the more bent over your posture is, the harder it is to get turned, or fully coiled, behind the ball. Your hips and shoulders can't rotate internally on the backswing; therefore, it's virtually impossible to swing the club in a rotary fashion. With limited mobility in your hips, and little to no rotation, you have to recruit the larger muscles in your upper body (shoulders, chest) to create power. On the downswing, your upper body will feel as though it has to move first, which it does, throwing the

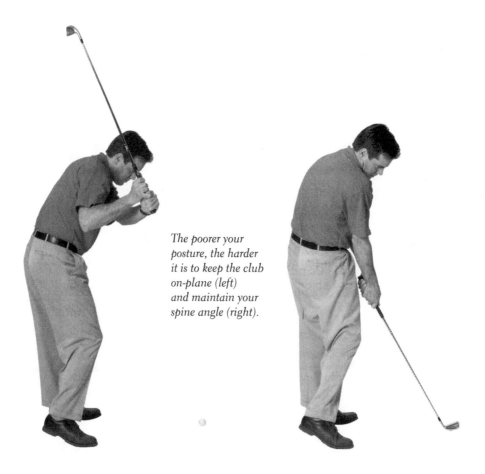

The poorer your posture, the harder it is to keep the club on-plane (left) and maintain your spine angle (right).

club on a steep, outside-to-in path, not the inside path you need to release the club and hit the ball solidly.

Maintaining good posture is a lifetime effort, one that gets more challenging as we get older. So how do you prevent your posture from sabotaging your swing and completely ruining your game? Here are a few pointers to help combat the forces of aging and keep your posture functional enough so that you can still put a good swing on the ball.

Brush Up On the Basics

The first thing you should do is see your golf pro or get in front of a mirror and review the fundamentals of good posture. These are a few basics to live by:

- Make sure your weight is evenly distributed over the balls of your feet, not out on your toes or back on your heels.
- Tilt your upper body forward from your hip joints, not your waist, so that your chest points toward the ground. All of your weight-bearing joints—top of your spine, inside of your elbows, front of your kneecaps, and balls of your feet—should form a straight line. "Picture yourself standing on a balance beam," says GOLF Magazine Top 100 Teacher Martin Hall. "To prevent yourself from falling off, you have to balance these joints out. Leaning too far back [on your heels] or too far forward [on your toes] will knock you off the beam."
- Add just enough knee flex so your kneecaps are over the balls of your feet.
- Your back should look fairly straight, not rounded. Feel as if your chest is tall and your shoulder blades are pinched toward each other.
- Tilt your upper body slightly away from the target so that your right shoulder is lower than your left, mirroring the position of your right hand on the grip (for a right-handed golfer).
- Allow your arms to hang naturally from your shoulders, like a rope with plenty of slack. If they're too tight (i.e., the rope is pulled taut), you're standing too far from the ball.

- To help check your distance from the ball, see that the butt of the club points toward your belt buckle (with a midiron); it will point slightly lower for a driver and slightly higher for a wedge.
- Keep your chin up; do not bury it in your chest.
- Adjust your feet so your stance is widest with a driver and narrowest with a wedge.

Stand at Attention

If you find yourself glued to the couch on the weekend, watching golf or some other sporting event, take a time-out and stand up. Place both hands behind the small of your back, applying very gentle pressure to your spine, and pinch your shoulder blades back toward each other, so you resemble a soldier standing at attention. Hold the pose for five minutes. This little exercise strengthens the back and shoulder muscles that are prone to fatigue in your setup, so that your upper body doesn't slouch over the ball. Hold this pose for several minutes each day and you'll have an easier time maintaining your posture throughout your swing. It also serves as a good reminder as to what the proper posture should feel like.

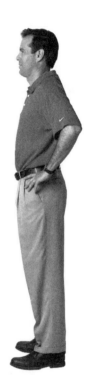

Make Some Alterations to Your Setup

It's very difficult for some golfers, particularly seniors, to hold their spine straight and maintain their posture for an entire swing. If your posture is in need of many repairs, and it can't be improved much, there are still some tweaks you can make to your setup to get your swing back on the right path. If you're having a hard time turning your hips in your backswing, flare out your back foot some. "This will give your hips more freedom to move so you can make a better turn behind the ball," says Brian Crowell, head teaching professional at GlenArbor Golf Club in Bedford Hills, New York. Conversely, Crowell says, if you're having a tough time swinging to a complete finish, you should flare your front foot out at address. Turning your front foot out makes it easier to clear your left hip out of the way, so your arms have room to swing down and your right side can release on through.

Another thing you can do is alter your grip. Many golfers, as they get older, turn their right hand over the top of the grip because it feels stronger to them. In reality,

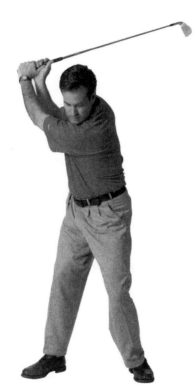

Flare your back foot out to turn your right hip more.

they are weakening their grip and promoting a very steep backswing plane. If they turn the right hand clockwise so it rests more under the shaft, they can swing the club more around their body, says Crowell. It may feel weaker, but it will add some pop to their drives because the club will be more likely to swing down from inside, not steep and across.

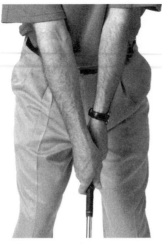
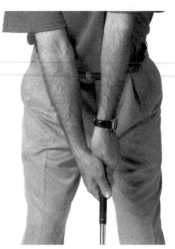

Weak Grip   *Strong Grip*

Keep Your Chin Up

Poor vision can also do harm to your posture. Many seniors, as their vision begins to deteriorate, adjust their heads so they're looking straight down at the ball. This forces

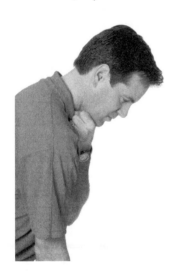

them to hunch over the ball, which drops their chin into their chest. If your chin is buried in your chest, there's little room to turn your shoulders back so you can get adequately behind the ball. Your shoulders get locked, which forces you to pick the club up and get too choppy with your swing.

Always keep some distance—at least a full fist, or the width of an orange—between your chin and your sternum, says Crowell. By keeping your chin up, your shoulders can turn freely to the top, which makes it easier to drop the club to the inside on the correct downswing path.

Change What's in Your Bag

As you get older and your flexibility and strength begin to wane, your game faces some new challenges: 1) Your swing speed diminishes; 2) you struggle more to get shots airborne; 3) your 250-yard drives become 200-yard drives; and 4) many of your clubs hit the ball the same distance. The good news is that with today's modern technology, you don't have to suffer significant losses in clubhead speed and yardage. If you adjust your set makeup to adapt to your strengths and weaknesses, you can still remain fairly competitive and long off the tee. As a matter of fact, with today's big-headed drivers and high-launch, low-spin golf balls, you can have a lot more fun than you had twenty years ago.

What clubs should be in your bag? Here are several things you can do to your set makeup to help you improve your game:

1. Replace your mid- and long-irons with hybrid clubs. With the weight concentrated farther from the clubface, it's much easier to get the ball airborne with these clubs, even with slower swing speeds.

2. Use graphite shafts only. The lightweight, flexible shafts will prevent you from losing too much clubhead speed.

3. Make sure your driver has at least 13 degrees of loft. Just because Tiger Woods swings an 8.5-degree driver doesn't mean you should. With your slower clubhead speed, you need the additional loft to launch the ball up into the air, which will improve your carry distance.

4. Don't switch to longer shafts, thinking that they will give you more power. The longer the club, the harder it is to control. Find something you can swing easily and in balance, because that will keep you in the fairway more often, which is the name of the game.

Aging is a natural process. It's like Tiger Woods with a fifty-four-hole lead in a golf tournament—unstoppable. But just because you're getting older doesn't mean your best golf is behind you. You can still learn to hit the ball farther and straighter if you work at it and remain in good physical condition. But if you don't stretch and exercise the appropriate golf muscles, and you allow your weight to balloon and your diet to deteriorate, you will compound the adverse effects of aging and speed up the process. Here are two important things to consider.

Watch Your Weight

Too much meat on your bones only accelerates the progression of the degenerative cascade, or wearing out of the tendons, joints, and disks in your body. The more load you put on these parts, the faster they wear out. It's like driving a heavier vehicle: If you're carrying around more weight, you need a higher grade of shock absorbers. Unfortunately, as we get older, these shocks are harder to manufacture.

Watch what you eat. Cut back on alcohol consumption and foods high in trans fats and saturated fats. Add more fruits, whole grains, and vegetables to your diet. Drink less soda and more water, and don't smoke. Cigarette smoking decreases blood supply to your tendons and disks, making them more susceptible to degeneration.

Work Your Core

Following the exercise routines outlined in *Golf Rx* will not only improve your golf performance and prevent injuries, but it will also help you to combat the damaging effects that aging can have on your posture. A strong midsection is needed to provide support for your upper torso, and *Golf Rx* targets the core muscles to give you this support so that your posture can remain more upright. There are also plenty of exercises to build strength and muscle endurance, as well as increase flexibility, so that you keep muscle loss and disk degeneration to a minimum.

CHAPTER FOUR

POWER EXERCISES TO STRETCH OUT YOUR DRIVES

In 1980, the first year the PGA Tour tracked individual statistics, the average driving distance on tour was 256.7 yards. Leading the way at 274.3 yards per pop was Dan Pohl, who won't be confused with John Daly anytime soon.

Today, if you averaged 274.3 yards on tour, you'd be considered a "short" hitter. You might even be asked to wear a skirt, as Fred Funk was, at the 2005 Skins Game after LPGA star Annika Sorenstam outdrove him on one hole. In 2005 alone, twenty-six players on the PGA Tour averaged 300 yards or better off the tee, led by Scott Hend at 318.9 yards. And it was even more out of hand on the Nationwide Tour, the PGA Tour's developmental tour. Forty-two players bested 300 yards, spearheaded by Bubba Watson, who at 334 yards nearly nuked each tee ball the length of 3½ football fields. It's no wonder Tiger Woods jokes about one day playing a hole that measures 900 yards, just to keep up with the length of today's heavy hitters. Not even the 650-yard 17th hole at Baltusrol Golf Club could tame Tiger in 2005—he hit the green during the final round of the PGA Championship with a driver and a 2-iron. Six hundred and fifty yards!

Professional golf has become a power game. Tour players bomb it as far as they can, not worried about whether or not they find the rough off the tee (because they'll have a short club in, anyway). There's still some finesse and shotmaking involved, but if you can't drive it far, you're at a serious disadvantage. Much of it is due to technology: Clubs are not only bigger, they're lighter, and they've been designed in such a way to optimize ball flight, ball speeds, and distance. But equally responsible for the big power surge is the attention these elite players are giving to physical fitness. Today's players work about as much on their bodies as they do on their swings.

Paul Schueren, a licensed physical therapist with both the PGA and Champions tours, estimates that more than half of the field will visit one of the PGA Tour's two on-site fitness trailers at least once during the course of a tournament. Schueren said that when he started with the Champions Tour in the late 1980s, a few curiosity seekers would stop by and peek their heads in, but today the trailers are often so crowded that players have to wait to use them.

The playing public has yet to grasp the importance of physical fitness, but they're starting to catch on. They see a chiseled Tiger or Vijay Singh hitting balls into the clouds, and they want to know their power secrets. They will do almost anything to outdrive their buddies. It's always nice to sink a twenty-foot putt for birdie, but there's no feeling quite like that of putting a big charge into a tee shot and sending one thirty or forty yards by your playing partners' longest drives.

The exercises that follow in this chapter won't have you outhitting Tiger anytime soon, but they will add some air-time and distance to your drives. I know because many of them are being performed daily in the PGA Tour fitness trailers and in the personal gyms of the best players in the world. They'll help you build a stronger core and more flexibility and clubhead speed, while also improving endurance so you're less prone to fatigue and injury.

(WARNING: Many of these exercises are advanced and involve weights and other training aids. Make sure to stretch and warm up adequately before attempting any of these movements, and check with your physical trainer or a fitness expert if you're unsure about how to perform any of these exercises properly.)

EXPLOSIVE SWING DRILL

"If you want to be fast, you have to train fast," says Scott Riehl, a physical therapist with the PGA Tour. "It's like training a runner to be a sprinter. You have to train the muscles to be quick. You're not training them to run the New York City Marathon."

One excellent way to do this is to find a club or training stick that is approximately 15 percent lighter than your average club and swing it, making sure to maintain your balance all the way into the finish. (You should be able to hold your finish for a count of five seconds.) Start with eight sets of three repetitions the first week, swinging at 60 percent of your max. Gradually increase the speed each week until you're swinging at about 110 percent. "The goal is to teach your body to move

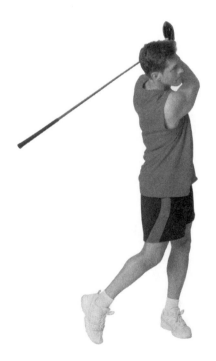

quicker and more explosively," says Jon Doyle, a strength and conditioning coach based in Fairfield County, Connecticut. "You want your last rep to be as explosive, or more so, than the first. When using high reps this is impossible. Each rep should be meaningful and purposeful."

Try This: Take your driver and turn it upside down, so that the clubhead is in your hands and the handle is closest to the ground. Then swing away. Because there's no weight on the end of the club, the handle will incur some resistance from the air as you swing. This will force you to accelerate your arms and body all the way into the finish, creating more clubhead speed.

Stand up straight with your feet about shoulder-width apart. Grab both ends of a resistance band or some stretchable tubing, with both elbows bent at 90 degrees. Keep both elbows nailed to your side as you turn your right forearm out, stretching the tubing. Slowly return your arm back to the starting position. Perform two sets of fifteen repetitions on each arm, three times per week, to strengthen the rotator cuff muscles in your shoulders.

Try This: At the end of the stretch, cup your right wrist backward so your knuckles move toward your forearm. This additional movement helps stretch the wrist extensors on the top of each forearm.

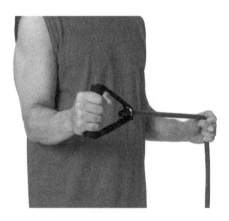

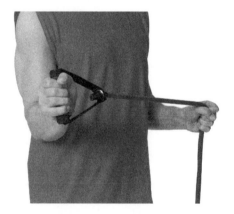

JACKKNIFE

Here's another golf-specific lower-abdominal exercise. Assume a push-up position with your feet and shins on an exercise ball. Your palms should be flat on the floor and your hands directly under your shoulders. Pull the ball forward, with your legs toward your chest, until your knees are in a straight line with your hips. This will bring your hips up toward the ceiling. Try to keep your head in line with your spine and do not let your hips sag toward the floor. Hold the contraction for two to three seconds, then return to the starting position. Perform two sets of fifteen reps, three times per week.

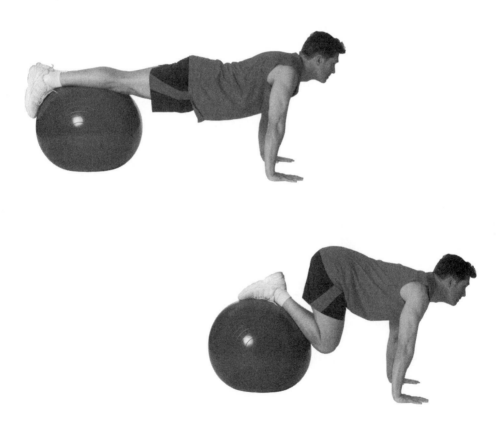

Stand in your normal golf posture with your right side facing a cable machine. Grab the handle at about shoulder height and pull the cable down diagonally toward the floor, rotating your trunk to the left just as you would if you were hitting a golf ball. Stop when your hands are just outside your left hip, and hold for a few seconds. Then slowly return the cable to the top, maintaining your posture throughout the entire movement—knees slightly flexed, chin up, back straight. Choose a weight that will allow you to perform fifteen reps. Perform two sets of fifteen reps, three times per week. If you don't have access to a gym, find some stretchable tubing or an elastic band and secure that to a door or other fixed object. Because you're mimicking the swing, this exercise incorporates all of the muscles in the swing, and helps strengthen and stabilize your core.

Try This: Repeat the exercise as above, but with your left side facing a cable machine or door. This way, you are mimicking a left-handed swing and increasing the strength and flexibility of your nondominant side.

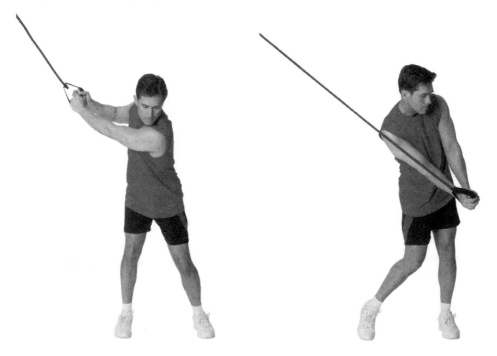

MED BALL THROW

Another good resistance exercise that mimics the golf swing is the med ball throw. Stand with your left side facing a wall or a partner. Hold a five-pound medicine ball in front of you just like you would a golf club, and make a backswing. Then rotate back to your left, shifting your weight onto your front leg, and fire the ball toward the wall. Do not release the ball too soon or you'll throw it straight into the ground. Your arms should be extended and your body facing the target as you throw. Perform two sets of fifteen reps, three times per week. Be careful not to exceed more than five pounds; you want just enough weight to create some resistance to your throwing motion. This exercise targets your entire core—abs, hips, lower back, and legs—increasing your rotational speed on the downswing.

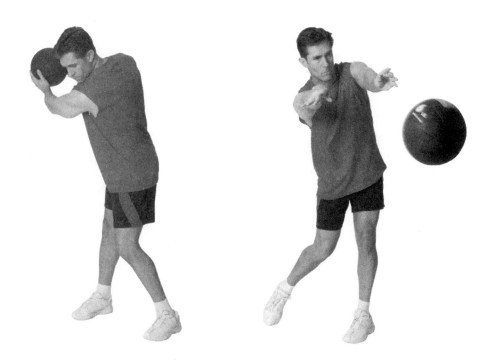

Hold a five-pound med ball or similar weight in front of your chest. Lunge forward with your right leg, slowly lowering your left knee until it's about two inches from the floor. Keep your back straight, and don't allow your right knee to extend past your toes. Hold the forward lunge for a count of one, and then rotate your shoulders to the right until the ball is directly in line with your right hip. Hold again for a count of one, and then rotate the ball back to center before returning to your starting position. Repeat with your left leg, twisting your torso to the left. Do two sets of ten reps on each side. The lunge portion of the exercise provides a great workout for your legs and glutes, while the twist strengthens your obliques and creates more range of motion in your torso.

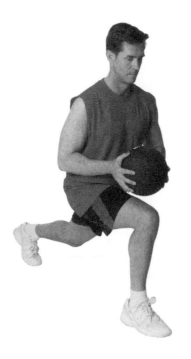 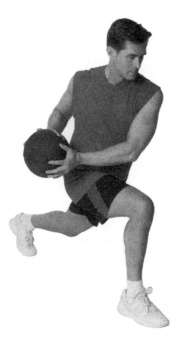

TORSO TWIST WITH CLUB

In the early 1990s, renowned instructor Jim McLean made headlines with his "X-Factor" swing theory. In simple terms, McLean's theory stated that if you turn your shoulders much farther than your hips in the backswing, you will hit the ball farther. The bigger the gap between the two, the more torque and resistance you create in the backswing, and the more explosive power you're able to generate in the downswing.

Here's a great exercise to stretch the "X." Sit on a stool or an exercise ball with a club lodged behind your lower back. Slowly rotate your right shoulder behind you until your left arm is directly in front of you and you feel a comfortable stretch in your back. Place your left hand on your left thigh to assist you in the rotation, and keep your pelvis facing forward. Hold for a count of five deep breaths in and out, then repeat on the opposite side. Perform three reps on each side, three times per week.

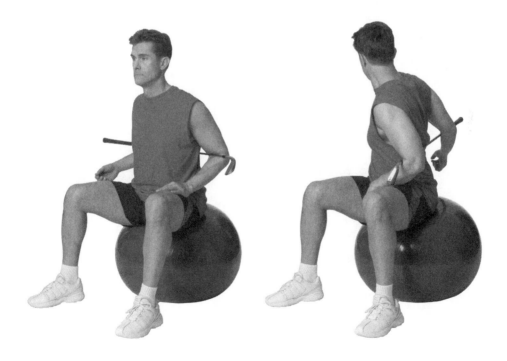

Lie on your back with your feet and calves resting on top of a stability ball and your legs bent at 90 degrees to your pelvis. Extend both arms at your side (palms down) for balance, and secure the ball tight into your glutes. Rotate your knees to one side, as far as your range of motion will allow. Hold the stretch for two to three seconds, then repeat on the other side. Do three sets of twelve reps. Keep both shoulders on the ground and your chest facing the ceiling throughout each movement. This exercise targets the hip external rotators and oblique muscles, which allow the torso to twist from side to side.

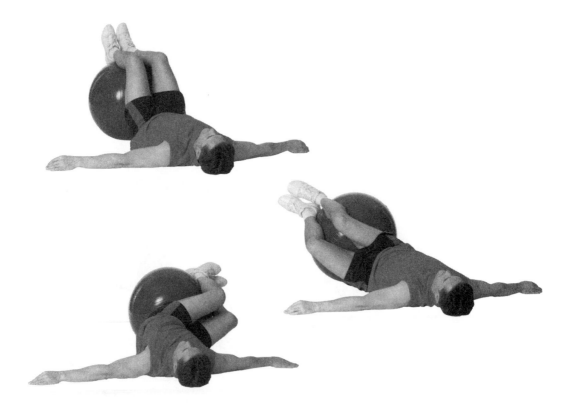

RUSSIAN TWIST ON BALL

Lie on a stability ball so your upper back and shoulders are supported by the ball and your hips are parallel to the floor, knees bent at 90 degrees. Hold a medicine ball or dumbbell straight over your chest and roll your shoulders to the left until your arms are parallel to the floor. Rotate back to center and then to the right, keeping your arms extended and your hips contracted upward, toward the ceiling (do not let them sag toward the floor). As you rotate from side to side, allow the ball to move with you, and try to keep your knees, hips, and chest in a straight line, parallel to the floor. Perform twelve reps on each side. This is one of the best abdominal exercises you can do because it targets both your internal and external obliques.

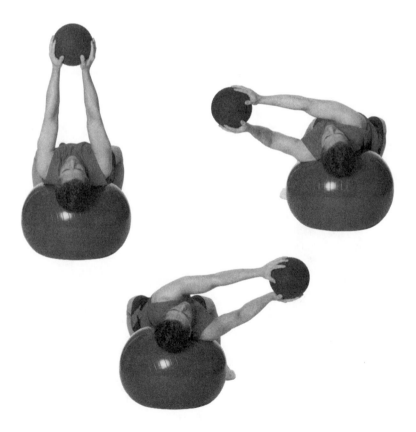

Start with a golf club (driver) before advancing on to a barbell or weights. Grab the club at both ends and extend it over your head so that both arms are locked and your hands are about 1½ times your shoulder-width apart. Stand up straight with your feet slightly wider than shoulder width, and then slowly go into a squat position, pushing your hips back so your butt moves toward the floor. Keep your elbows locked, your eyes looking forward, and your chest up during the movement. Squat down until you start to feel your posture slipping, and then return to the starting position. Perform six sets of four repetitions or eight sets of three, but do not exceed twenty-four reps. This exercise works just about every major muscle in the golf swing—glutes, hips, upper back (rhomboids), shoulders—building strength, speed, and endurance.

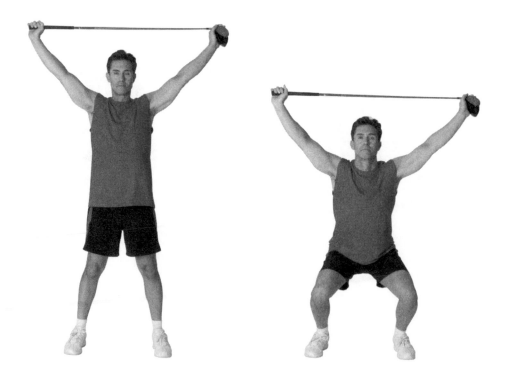

WINDMILL

Grasp a long iron or driver midshaft with your right hand, and extend your right arm straight up toward the sky so the shaft is parallel to the ground. Stand with your feet slightly wider than your shoulders, your right foot pointed in about 45 degrees and your left foot flared out 90 degrees. Keeping your right leg straight and left leg slightly bent, push your hips back toward your right leg and bend forward in the opposite direction until your left hand touches the ground—or your left foot. At this point, your arms and shoulders should form a straight line, like a windmill. Fix your eyes on the overhead hand throughout the entire movement, and keep the number of reps low (no more than eight reps on each side). When the exercise becomes easier, switch to a heavier barbell. This exercise increases flexibility in your core, stretches your obliques, glutes, and hamstrings, and stabilizes your shoulders.

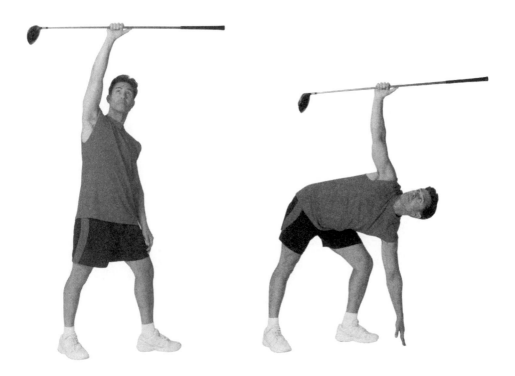

Lie facedown on the floor with your feet and elbows shoulder-width apart and your palms flat on the floor. Draw your abdominals in and raise your hips and torso off the floor, using your forearms and toes for support. Your hips and shoulders should form a straight line, or bridge; do not allow your hips to sag toward the floor. Hold this "plank" position for thirty seconds, then repeat twice more. As the exercise gets easier, increase the time to sixty seconds. This is another terrific core-strengthening exercise because it targets the deepest of the abdominal muscles—the transverse abdominals—and the paraspinals.

Try This: To work your inner abdominals even harder, lift one leg off the ground while you're in the plank position (*bottom photo*).

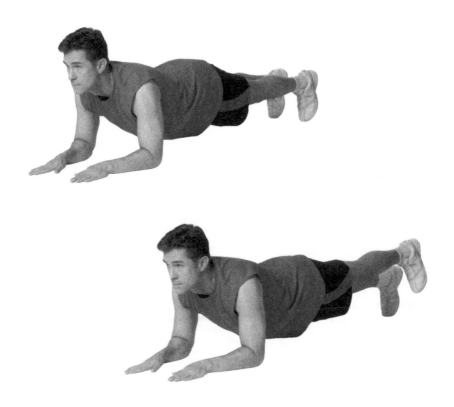

SIDE PLANK

Lie on your right side with your weight supported by your right elbow and your arms, hips, and legs in a straight line. Lift your body off the ground to form a plank, balancing your weight on your forearm and the side of your foot. Tighten your abs and buttocks to keep your body in a straight line, and try to relax your shoulders. Hold this position for thirty seconds and switch sides, putting your weight on your left arm and elbow. Repeat twice more on both sides. In addition to strengthening your core abdominal muscles, this exercise helps stabilize your shoulders and back.

Try This: Lift your top leg in a scissor-like motion—fast on the way up, slow on the way down—to strengthen your hip abductor muscles. Targeting these muscles will help you generate more clubhead speed.

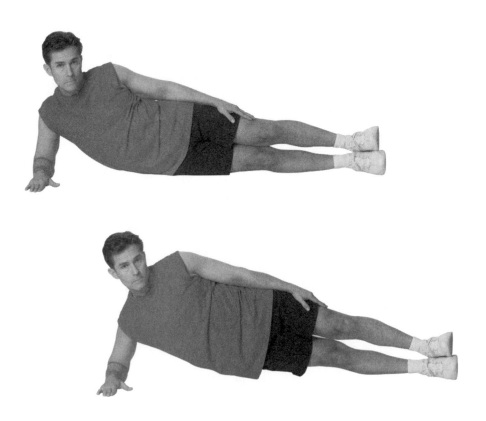

In order to swing the club efficiently and with maximum speed, you need to rotate your trunk around a stable base, or platform, says Vern McMillan, personal trainer to a number of top Australian players on the PGA Tour, including Adam Scott and Stuart Appleby. "Power is created from the ground up. If you can't impart force [on the ball] from below your core, then you'll try and impart force farther up," says McMillan. "Your joints and muscles get smaller as you move toward your fingers, and they're not designed to handle that type of load."

A good way to train the body to move in the most efficient manner is to set up in your normal golf posture with your right foot extended in front of your left—as though you were taking a big stride forward with your right foot. Bend from your hips and extend both arms in front of you so that your hands are in front of your knees. Rotate your arms back and through as far as your range of motion will allow, maintaining your posture (this is key) and the triangle formed by your arms and shoulders. Change legs after ten repetitions. To create additional resistance and engage your core muscles even more, hold on to a five-pound med ball as you perform each movement (*photos, opposite page*), rotating the ball from side to side just as if you were making a golf swing.

Congratulations! You've taken a big step toward outdriving your buddies off the tee. Perform these exercises regularly, as well as the strengthening and endurance exercises in Series B and C (Chapters Thirteen and Fourteen), and it won't be long before you're driving your ball to places in the fairway you've never seen before, and hitting shorter clubs into the greens. Now, to learn how to stretch properly before and after a round, and to keep loose during the round so you can fully reap the benefits of your newfound power, proceed on to Chapters Five through Seven.

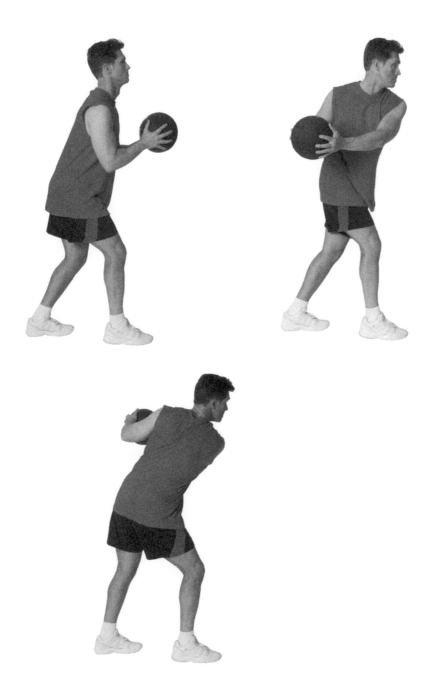

CHAPTER FIVE

PREGAME:
A FIVE-MINUTE WARM-UP PROGRAM

Your car screeches to a halt in the parking lot, tires burning, only fifteen minutes prior to your regular Saturday-morning tee time. That leaves you just enough time to check in, warm up, and head to the first tee. Granted, it's not enough time to prepare for eighteen holes of golf—ideally, you want to arrive forty-five minutes to an hour before teeing off, enough time to stretch, hit a few balls on the practice range, and hit some putts—but it will have to do on this day.

Many golfers would take the five minutes they have and proceed directly to the practice green, or even the range, to get in a few final licks. But that's no way to get your body ready for four-plus hours of repeated golf swings. You're only asking for trouble, perhaps even a serious injury that will keep you off the course for weeks or months to come.

Think about it: Unless you're a professional golfer, you probably spent the entire week sitting behind a desk, your body in a shortened, bent position for eight to ten hours each day. Now you're asking your body to go into extension, to be extremely limber and explosive so you can pound a golf ball for the next four-plus hours. That just doesn't happen by showing up. You have to stretch and restore some elasticity to your hips, back, shoulders, hamstrings, and other golf-specific muscles, so that they can perform the movements you're about to ask of them.

Here are five exercises you should do before each round or practice routine to raise the temperature and readiness of these muscles. Perform each exercise standing, since that is how you'll be conducting your business for the next four-plus hours. The warm-up should only take five minutes, a suitable time frame for those of you who do tend to run a little late.

STANDING SHOULDER/BACK STRETCH

Stand up straight with your arms at your sides and your feet shoulder-width apart. Bring your right arm out in front of your chest and place the back of your left hand, palm facing forward, against your forearm. Straighten your right arm and gently pull it toward your chest with your left hand, stretching it all the way out. Stop when you feel a good stretch at the back of your right shoulder, and hold for at least five deep breaths in and out. Switch arms and repeat, using your right hand to pull your left arm across your chest. This exercise stretches the posterior shoulder capsules and

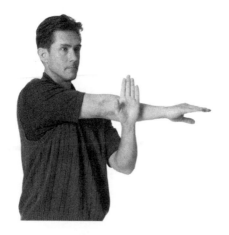 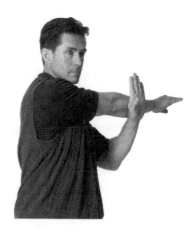

muscles, including the rear deltoids, and your lower back muscles, promoting an efficient turn behind the ball.

FIGURE-FOUR STRETCH

From a standing position, cross your right leg over your left so that your legs form a figure four. Squat down into your left hip and, using your right hand, push down on your right knee (toward the floor) until you feel a good stretch in your right glute. Hold for at least five deep breaths in and out and then repeat on the other leg. Should you struggle to keep your balance, hold on to a golf club or a cart with your free hand to offer better support (*below*). This is commonly known as a standing "FABERE" stretch—FABERE is an acronym for Flexion, ABduction, External Rotation, and Extension. In addition to the glutes, this exercise stretches your hip flexors and abductors, improving your overall stability and increasing the range of motion in your hips.

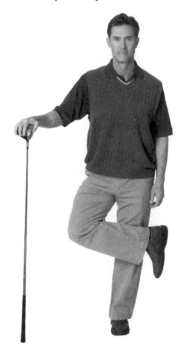 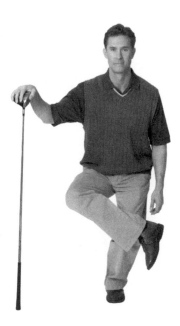

Stand as though you were about to address a ball, bending slightly forward from your hips so your chest points toward the ground. Your back should be fairly straight and your knees flexed. Loop your forearms around a club, holding the shaft gently against your back. Now, slowly rotate your hips and shoulders to the right, until your right arm is directly behind you. Hold for at least five deep breaths in and out, then slowly twist in the other direction until your left arm is behind you. Hold again for five deep breaths, then repeat. Perform up to three repetitions, but no more. This exercise targets the paraspinal muscles, which run up and down each side of your spine. Besides stabilizing the spine, these muscles act like pistons, transferring energy generated by your legs to your arms.

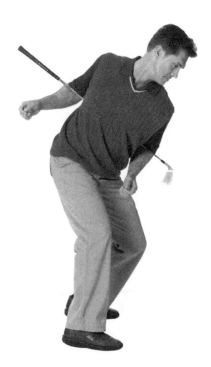

HAMSTRING/CALF STRETCH

Stand with your right leg forward (knee bent) and your left leg extended back in a straight position. Slowly lean forward into your right leg, keeping your left leg straight and both feet flat on the floor. Stop when your right knee is over the shoelaces on your right foot, and hold for at least thirty seconds. Repeat with your opposite leg, keeping your back straight as you lunge forward. This exercise stretches your calves and hamstrings, freeing up your hips while also providing support to your back in the deceleration phase of the swing.

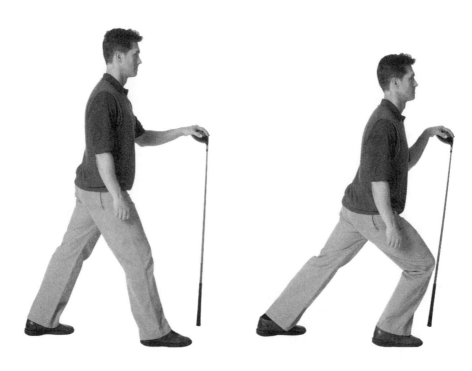

Lean slightly forward from your hips and extend your left arm straight out in front of you for better balance. Next, grab your right foot with your right hand and gently pull your foot up toward your right glute. The farther you pull your knee back, the deeper you stretch your hip-flexor muscle. Hold the stretch for five deep breaths in and out, then switch legs. Try and keep both knees close together while performing this stretch. This is an important stretch, because the average golfer spends most of the workday in a hip flexor–shortened position—what I refer to in Chapter Two as the "desk-job syndrome." If you don't stretch these muscles out, you will tend to bend over too much, severely limiting your ability to turn your shoulders and maintain your posture throughout the swing.

Now, go play some golf. If time permits, hit a few putts and chips before heading to the first tee. Having stretched your golf-specific core muscles, you should feel limber, relaxed, and more confident for your round.

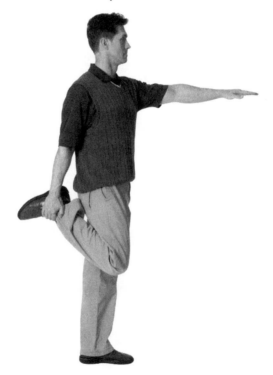

CHAPTER SIX

TEE TO GREEN: EIGHTEEN STRETCHES FOR EIGHTEEN HOLES

In the four-plus hours it normally takes to play a round of golf, you will spend only a fraction of the time hitting balls or mentally preparing to do so. Most of the time, you'll be walking to your ball or waiting for someone else in your group to play, or waiting on the group in front of you to clear. At times, you'll feel like you're sitting in traffic on the expressway, patiently waiting for the logjam in front of you to exit.

Because golf is such a mental game, what you do with this time can largely impact your performance on the course. LPGA Hall of Famer Annika Sorenstam doesn't waste this time—she likes to "go on vacation" between shots. She will talk to one of her playing partners, hum a song to herself, or think about how she wants to redecorate a room back home. She doesn't spend all of her time thinking about the shot ahead or beating herself up over the one she just hit in the rough. To do that for four-plus hours would be exhausting. She tries hard to stay in the moment, and taking the occasional vacation helps her do just that.

Another great way to "go on vacation" is to use this time to stretch. Not only will this put your mind at ease, but it will keep your body loose and limber, which is essential when you're asking it to apply the accelerator and brakes so much. You need endurance for those last few holes, because a tired, stiff body is very prone to injury and bad shots.

Here are eighteen stretches you can do—one for each hole of the course—as you wait.

HOLE ONE: NECK STRETCH

From a standing position, slowly turn your chin to the left so it's in line with your left shoulder. Place your right palm on your left cheek and gently push your head in the opposite direction—toward your right shoulder. Hold for a count of five deep breaths in and out, and repeat on the other side. Keep your shoulders relaxed and your chest facing forward as you rotate your head. This exercise stretches the muscles

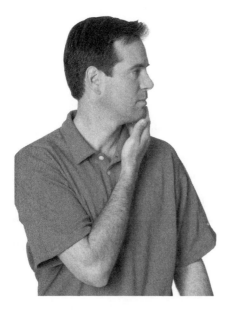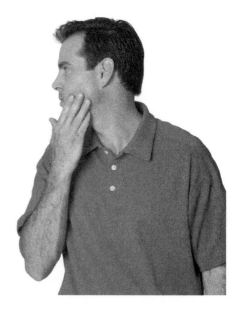

in the back of your neck, which is very important to controlling the motion of your head during the swing.

Bonus Tip: You can stretch your pecs (chest muscles), too, by putting your left arm directly behind you as you turn your head to the right. Put your right arm behind you when rotating your chin to the left.

HOLE TWO: SHOULDER STRETCH

Slide your right hand underneath your left armpit and grab your back, just under your left shoulder blade. Do the same with your left hand, latching on to your right shoulder blade. Next, pull your shoulders back as far as you can, as if you were trying to get each arm to touch the opposite shoulder blade. Hold for a count of five deep breaths in and out. This exercise strengthens the rhomboid muscles in the middle of your back, which are responsible for stabilizing and pinning the shoulder blades back. They help to give you the straight-back look that is so important to holding your posture throughout the swing.

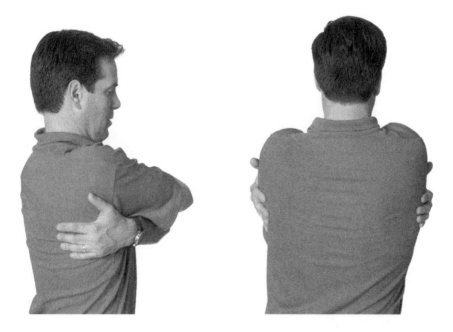

Hold your right arm straight out in front of you with your palm facing outward and fingers pointing toward the sky. Using your left hand, gently pull back the fingers of your right hand, toward your forearm. Hold for a count of five deep breaths in and out, then switch arms. You should feel a stretch on the underside of each forearm, in your wrist-flexor muscles.

To stretch the wrist extensors at the top of your forearm, hold your right arm out in front of you with your palm facing you and fingers pointing toward the ground. With your left hand, gently pull your fingers toward you until you feel a good stretch on top of your arm (*below*). Hold for a count of five deep breaths in and out. Besides keeping your wrists supple, both exercises will help to avoid such common elbow injuries as golfer's elbow (tendinitis on the inside of the elbow) and tennis elbow (tendinitis on the outside of the elbow).

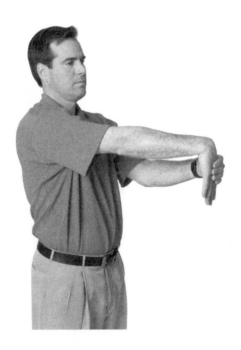

HOLE FOUR: PEC STRETCH A

Grip both ends of a club and lift it up over your head, so that both of your arms are fully extended. Slowly pull the club back behind your head, keeping both elbows straight. Take the club back as far as your range of motion will allow without bending your elbows, and hold for a count of five deep breaths in and out. This exercise helps open up (i.e., lengthens) your chest muscles, or pecs, which get shortened very easily when you're sitting behind a desk or in front of a computer all day long. It also stretches your tricep muscles, promoting a fuller, more efficient turn behind the ball.

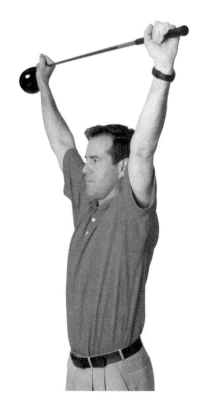 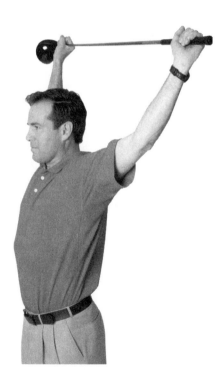

Hold a club (preferably a driver or longer club) behind your back, gripping it at both ends. Bend slightly forward from the hips and, keeping both arms fairly straight, bring the club up toward your neck. Hold for a count of five deep breaths in and out. You'll feel more of a stretch in your triceps on this exercise, in addition to your pecs, upper back, neck, and bicep muscles.

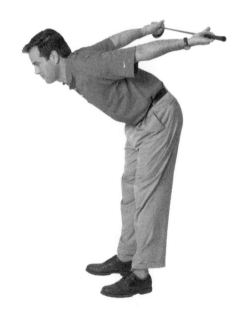

HOLE SIX: HAMSTRING/BACK STRETCH

This is a favorite exercise of five-time British Open champion Tom Watson. Stand up straight with your feet shoulder-width apart and your arms at your sides. Next, reach your right hand toward your left big toe while extending your left arm up toward the sky. Keep your legs straight and your neck relaxed. Hold for a count of at least thirty seconds. This is a great full-body exercise, because it stretches the paraspinals, hip rotators, hamstrings, and calves.

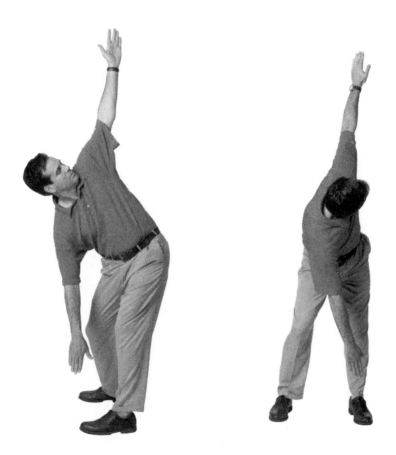

Take the longest club in your bag, your driver, and bring it out to your side so the clubhead sits in your left palm, and your right hand rests on top of the butt end of the grip. Your right arm should be fully extended, with the clubhead at approximately waist height.

Push up on the clubhead with your left palm until you feel a good stretch in your right side. The "high" hand should maintain a hold on the end, but should not push down on it. Keep the long arm relaxed and hold for a count of five deep breaths in and out. Repeat on the other side. This exercise, devised by Mike Shaw, an assistant teaching professional at Leewood Country Club in Eastchester, New York, targets your upper lat muscles to give you a fuller stretch in your backswing.

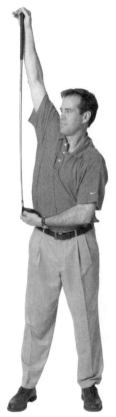

HOLE EIGHT: SIDE BEND WITH CLUB

Hold a club over your head with both arms extended wide. Bend to one side as far as your range of motion will allow, making sure to keep both elbows straight and your head centered, or equidistant from both arms. Hold for a count of five deep breaths in and out, and then return to the starting position. Repeat on the other side. You'll feel a good stretch in your obliques, and you'll also reap the benefits of improved posture.

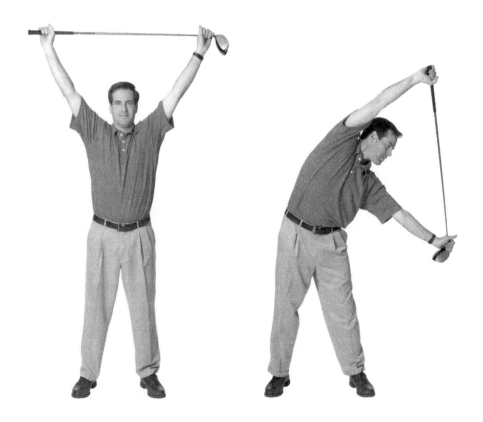

Hold a club out in front of you with both hands and cross your right leg over your left. Lower the club slowly toward the ground as far as you can go, bending from your hips, not your back. Keep your rear knee straight. Hold for five deep breaths in and out, then return to a standing position and repeat with your opposite leg. This is a good stretch for your hamstrings and paraspinals.

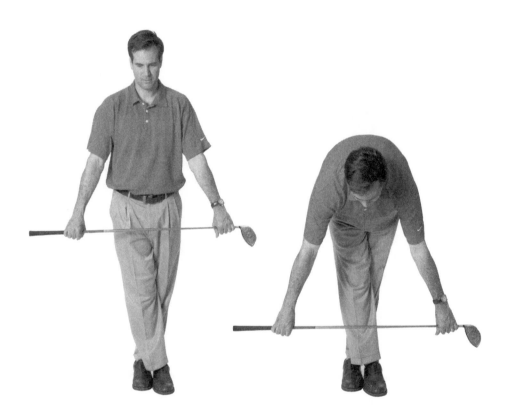

HOLE TEN: STANDING BACKWARD BEND

Stand erect with your knees slightly bent and your hands on your hips. Bend back slowly, lowering the base of your neck toward the ground. Look straight up at the sky as you arch your back as far as your range of motion will allow. You should feel a gentle stretch in your back (paraspinals) and abs. Hold for a count of five deep breaths in and out. WARNING: Pay strict attention to form and do not overextend your back.

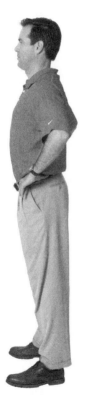
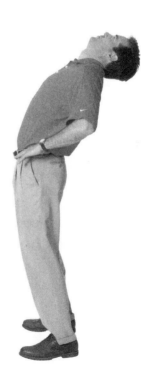

Stand with your left side facing a golf cart, wall, or something stable. You can even use a club for balance. Cross your right leg behind your left and lean your weight into your right hip, pushing it away from the cart. At the same time, let your upper body fall in the other direction, to the left, so you feel a good stretch in your right leg and hip. You're actually stretching a thick band of tissue called the iliotibial band (ITB) on the outside of your leg. Hold for five deep breaths in and out and repeat several more times before switching legs.

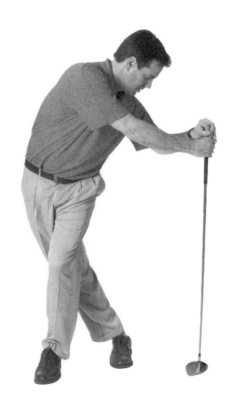

HOLE TWELVE: ITB STRETCH, 45 DEGREES

From a standing position, cross your left foot over your right and then slowly lower your hands toward the ground at a 45-degree angle to your starting position (90 degrees being straight ahead). Make sure to bend from your waist, then extend your arms as far as you can while maintaining good balance. Hold for a count of at least five deep breaths in and out, and repeat on the other leg. You should feel a good stretch in your outer thigh, obliques, and glutes.

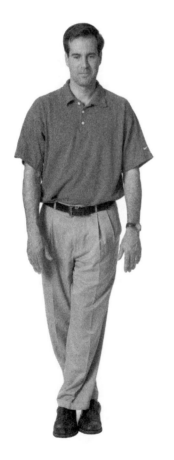
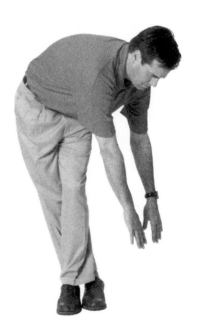

Stand with your feet shoulder-width apart and knees slightly bent. Place your hands on your waist and slowly turn from side to side, keeping your toes and knees facing forward and your back straight. As you rotate to your right side, try to get your right elbow behind you, and vice versa. Allow your head to turn naturally with your spine. This exercise will increase your torso flexibility and your ability to rotate back and through.

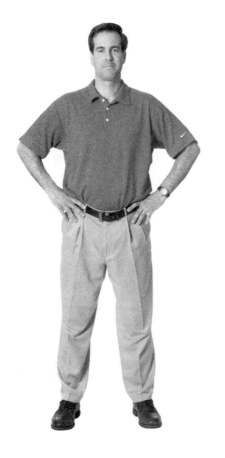
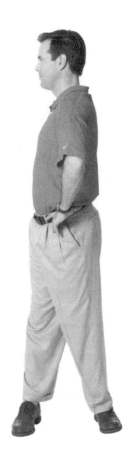

HOLE FOURTEEN: HIP-ABDUCTOR STRETCH (SINGLE LEG)

Stand erect with your feet shoulder-width apart and arms extended straight out in front of you for balance. Lift your right foot off the ground just enough to shift your weight onto your left leg, and kick your leg out to the right. Keep your knee straight and your body centered. Return to the starting position. Perform a set of ten reps on each leg to help strengthen your gluteal muscles and improve your lateral movement.

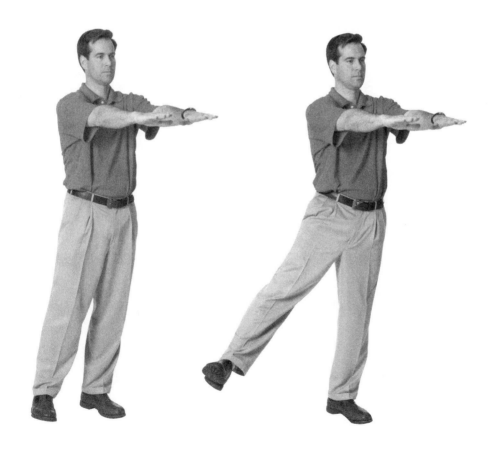

From a standing position, bend slightly forward from your hips. Bring your right knee up toward your chest and then grasp the back of your thigh with both hands. Without slumping forward, pull your knee up toward your body as high as your range of motion will allow. Hold for a count of five deep breaths in and out, and then return to the starting position. Repeat on the other leg to give your hip-flexor muscles a good stretch.

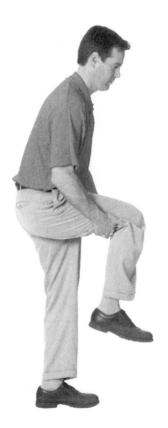
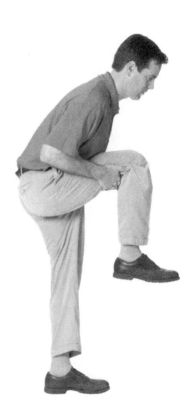

HOLE SIXTEEN: HIP-FLEXOR STRETCH WITH CART

Stand two to three feet away from the back of a golf cart (a bench will do if you're walking) and place your right foot up on the back of the cart. Extend your left leg behind you and lean into the cart, pushing your hips forward until you feel a good stretch at the front of your right hip. Squeeze your right buttock for a deeper stretch in the hip. Hold for a count of five deep breaths in and out and switch legs.

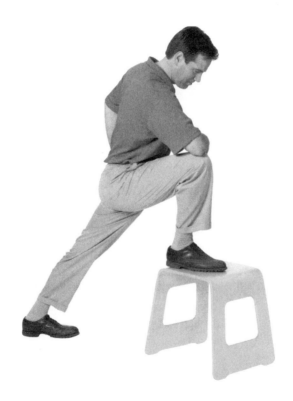

Lean against a wall, a golf cart, or other stationary object. Extend your right leg behind you with your heel flat on the ground. Your left leg should be bent and much closer to the wall. Lower your outstretched leg toward the ground and gently lean toward the wall, keeping your back fairly straight. Hold for a count of at least five deep breaths in and out, then switch legs. You should feel a good stretch in your lower calf muscles, which will help to improve your footwork and balance during the swing.

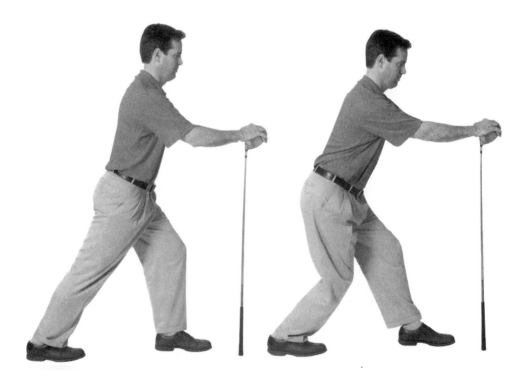

HOLE EIGHTEEN: ACHILLES/ANKLE STRETCH

From a standing position, cross your right leg in front of your left at a 45-degree angle so your legs form a figure four. Make sure your right heel is off the ground and the toes of your right foot are curled underneath you. Almost all of your weight should be distributed on your left leg.

Apply some pressure to your right calf with your left leg (tibia). This will bring your right foot forward, creating a stretch on the top half of your foot. Hold for a count of five deep breaths in and out and repeat on the other foot to stretch your ankle and Achilles tendon.

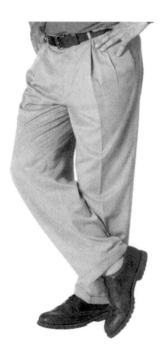 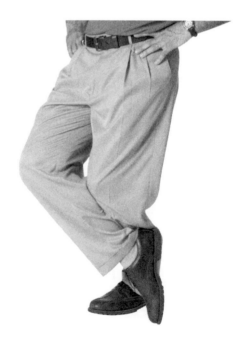

CHAPTER SEVEN

POSTGAME:
A FIVE-MINUTE COOLDOWN PROGRAM

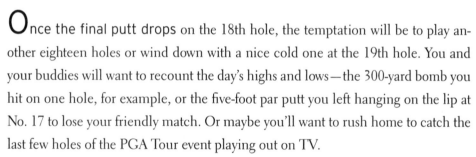

Once the final putt drops on the 18th hole, the temptation will be to play another eighteen holes or wind down with a nice cold one at the 19th hole. You and your buddies will want to recount the day's highs and lows—the 300-yard bomb you hit on one hole, for example, or the five-foot par putt you left hanging on the lip at No. 17 to lose your friendly match. Or maybe you'll want to rush home to catch the last few holes of the PGA Tour event playing out on TV.

There's nothing wrong with a little post-round fun and relaxation. Surely you earned the right to get off your feet for a while. But before you call it a day, take five minutes to stretch out your muscles and joints. You'll be happy you did, especially if you want to play eighteen holes the following day, because stretching immediately afterward helps combat muscle soreness and stiffness and keeps your body feeling supple and relaxed.

You don't have to stretch immediately, but you'll want to do so within forty-five minutes of your last stroke. This is your window of opportunity, a time when your core temperature is elevated and your muscles are warm and ready to be stretched safely. This is the goal of the cooldown: to stretch those muscles that need to be lengthened. Should you wait until you get home or leave it until the following morning, you will have squandered this opportunity and risked injury because your muscles won't be as warm and supple. Never stretch cold muscles. Always warm up before beginning any stretching or exercise routine, lightly jogging in place, going for a brisk walk, or riding a stationary bike to increase the temperature and flexibility of your muscles.

Here are five simple stretches you can do after your round, without even leaving the golf course. Best of all, you can do all but one of them in a seated position, because after standing for so long, you'll want to sit down. Find a dry patch of grass or an open, carpeted section in your locker room, and take a seat. These five exercises will not only improve your flexibility, they'll enhance your recovery time . . . just in case you do want to tee it up the following morning.

FINGERS TO TOES

From a seated position, extend both legs straight out in front of you with your toes pointed upward. Slowly bend forward and try to touch your toes with your finger-

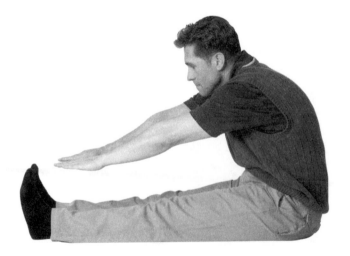

tips. Bend forward as far as your range of motion will allow, keeping your back as tall as possible. Do not hunch over. Hold for at least five deep breaths in and out and repeat twice more. This stretch improves your hamstring flexibility, so that you have an easier time bending from the hips and holding your address posture. It also opens up the facet joints in your back, reducing pressure on them so that the spine can move more freely.

SEATED ITB STRETCH

From a tall, seated position, cross your right leg over your left and extend your right arm behind you for support. Your right foot should rest flat on the floor, just to the outside of your left knee. Using your left arm, pull your right knee toward your left hip while rotating your torso slowly in the opposite direction. Keep turning your body until you can see the fingers on your right hand. Hold for a count of five deep breaths in and out and then repeat on the other side. This stretch targets the iliotibial band, a taut band of tissues on the outside of your thigh, paraspinals, gluteus medius, and hip abductors, which assist in rotating your hips externally.

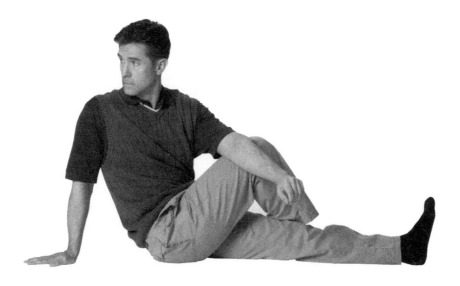

CROSS-LEGGED HIP STRETCH

Sit on the floor with legs crossed. Slowly bend forward from the waist and place both palms on the floor, keeping your elbows and back straight. Lean into the floor until you feel a good stretch in your hips and lower back. Hold for at least five deep breaths in and out. This is another good stretch for the hip flexors and facet joints of your back. It lengthens these joints and muscles, which sit in a shortened position most of the day.

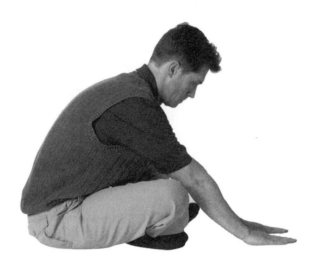

LYING BACK/HIP-FLEXOR STRETCH

Lie on your back with legs bent at 90 degrees and both feet off the floor. Slide your arms under both knees and clasp your hands together to form a chain. Now slowly pull your knees toward your chest with both arms and bring your head toward both knees. This should pull your shoulders off the ground. Hold the stretch for five deep breaths in and out and repeat twice more. This is another good exercise for tight hip flexors; it also helps lengthen the muscles and joints in your back.

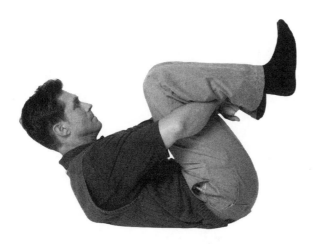

Sit tall on the ground in a butterfly position with the soles of your feet pressed together and both knees off the floor. Bend slightly forward from the waist and rest your hands on your lower legs. Now gently press your knees toward the floor with your elbows until you feel a good stretch along the inside of your thighs. Hold for at least five deep breaths in and out and repeat twice more. This exercise stretches the groin muscles located between your thigh and abdomen, improving your range of motion in your hip region so that you can make a fuller backswing.

Congratulations! You're finished with your post-round stretching routine. Now go enjoy a few beers with your buddies at the bar, or go out for a nice dinner. You'll feel as loose as you did on the 10th tee, so you'll be able to enjoy your post-round activities without your back tightening up or your muscles aching. Better yet, you'll be able to tee it up again in the morning and play another eighteen holes, should you feel up to it.

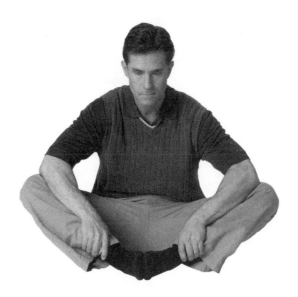

CHAPTER EIGHT

HOW TO WIN WITH
THE BODY YOU HAVE

There is a saying in golf that the ball doesn't know who you are. It doesn't matter if you're tall, short, thin, or stocky—it's a ball, and therefore it doesn't conspire or discriminate against you.

However, your body type does influence the way you swing a golf club. If you're six foot four, you'll be able to create a bigger swing arc and more clubhead speed than someone who is five-four, stocky, and not as flexible, but you'll also have a harder time getting down to the ball and maintaining your posture. There are advantages and disadvantages to being tall, short, lean, or barrel-chested. Which one are you? The following chapter will help you to identify which camp you fall into, what your natural tendencies are because of your body type, and how you can make it work for you.

In their book *The LAWs of the Golf Swing*, *GOLF Magazine* Top 100 Teachers Mike Adams, T. J. Tomasi, and Jim Suttie identify three different body types—leverage, arc, and width—which have become the standard by which golfers are typecast today. The leverage player is a classic *mesomorph*, or muscular type. If you fit this description, you are more athletic than most but have average flexibility. Your arms and legs are proportional in size, so your swing is more balanced and rotational than an arc or width player, and therefore requires the least amount of maintenance of the three. It is the simplest swing to repeat.

A good example of a leverage player today is Fred Funk, the 2005 winner of the Players Championship. There isn't a tremendous amount of hip rotation or burst in his swing, but his upper and lower body are very much in sync as they unwind through the ball. Perhaps that is why he is one of the most accurate drivers of the ball in the history of the game. Other leverage players today include LPGA Hall of Famer Annika Sorenstam, Sergio Garcia, Chris DiMarco, and Retief Goosen.

The leverage player generates his or her power through the hinging and unhinging of the wrists and the folding and unfolding—or straightening—of the arms. "They set levers and straighten levers," says Adams—and levers are multipliers of power.

The disadvantages to being a leverage player are minimal compared to an arc or width player. If there are any disadvantages, it's that they're not as flexible as the tall, lanky arc players, which makes them susceptible to shoulder and elbow injuries. For more on how to keep these parts limber, see the "Shoulder Stretch" and "Elbow and Wrist Stretch" in Chapter Six.

THE ARC PLAYER

The arc player, or *ectomorph*, is your tall, slender body type. This group tends to have long arms and terrific flexibility, and these players use their height advantage to generate power. Some good examples of arc players today include Davis Love III, Sean O'Hair, and, to a large degree, Michelle Wie. Tiger Woods, in his earlier years, was a classic ectomorph, although he is now more a hybrid of all three, having added significant muscle mass to his frame while also tightening his swing.

The advantage to being so long-limbed and flexible is that you have the wherewithal to create a lot of width in your swing. The wider the arc, the more distance the clubhead travels and the more speed and power you're able to generate. It's like a line of skaters moving around the ice in a circle: The skater closest to the center moves the least amount of distance and therefore travels at the slowest rate of speed, but the skater at the end covers the most ice and thus generates the most velocity.

Arc players also tend to be very languid, almost lazy, in their delivery of the club, says Tomasi. There's a gradual buildup of acceleration that is unleashed at impact as the right side catches the left and fires through, almost like a slinging or catapulting motion.

The disadvantage to being an arc player is that you're always trying to bulk up. Arc players often think of themselves as being too thin. They also tend to be very leggy on the downswing. The lower body gets overactive, and there is too much of a lateral shift of the hips on the forward swing. As a result, the lower body outraces the arms to the ball, and the player has to wait for the hands to catch up. It's very easy for an arc player to get the club stuck behind him or her, which can lead to a lot of errant shots—in particular, blocks and hooks.

Taller players are also more prone to back injuries, because they don't have the supportive muscle mass, and they need to bend more to get down to the ball. They're so flexible that they often rotate their bodies farther than they should, which puts additional strain on the facet joints in the back.

What the arc player could use is the more rotary motion that the leverage player exhibits. They should feel as though their upper body is turning over their lower body, says Tomasi, so that their arm-swing matches up better to their body turn.

Being very tall, there's also a tendency to make too upright a backswing, which leads to an overswinging of the arms. This significantly narrows the swing arc, thus negating any height advantage. To keep your arm-swing in check, feel as though your body and your arms reach the top at the same time. "Make sure your right arm doesn't bend more than 90 degrees at the top," says GOLF Magazine Top 100 Teacher Mike Bender, a former PGA Tour player. "To hit the ball far, you need to maintain a circular radius to your arc, like the spokes on a wheel. If you bend the right arm, you change the length of the spoke."

THE WIDTH PLAYER

The width player, or *endomorph*, is characterized by a thick chest, wide torso, and short arms. He has a stocky, almost box-like appearance, and is generally not very flexible. John Daly is a width player, yet he has tremendous flexibility, as evidenced by his enormous shoulder turn (more than 100 degrees) and clubhead position at the top of his swing—it nearly touches the ground. Daly is an exception to the rule, however. Some other examples of width players include Craig Stadler, Jason Gore, Duffy Waldorf, and Hal Sutton.

What these big guys lack in flexibility they make up for in strength. While they have very little flexibility in their hips, and their swings tend to be shorter and more compact (except Daly), they have tremendous upper-body strength, which can translate into big gains off the tee. A shorter arm-swing can also be an advantage: The less distance your hands and arms have to travel, the better your chances are of returning the clubface square at impact. As long as you clear your hips—creating room for the arms to swing down freely—and shift your weight properly, you can use your superior strength to power the ball a long way.

The disadvantage to being a width player is that because you have shorter arms, you have a shorter lever to work with, and you're therefore not able to generate as much width (of the arc) as the arc player is. Also, because your upper body is so strong, it will have a natural tendency to want to take over on the downswing. If the shoulders unwind before your lower body has a chance to, you will throw the club over the top on a steep, out-to-in path. This swing will feel more powerful (short and bursty), but it will actually cause you to lose clubhead speed, control, and distance.

Short, stocky endomorphs are also more susceptible to lower-body injuries—in particular, knees and hips—because of the additional weight being placed on these joints and tendons.

If you're a width player and your strength is not translating into extra yards, there are a few adjustments you can make to your setup to help, according to Tomasi. First, drop your right foot several inches back, away from the target line. This will create some space for your arms so you can drop the club into the slot—on an inside path—on the downswing. Second, flare, or turn, your right foot out some, which will allow you to turn your right hip more so you can make a bigger shoulder turn. And last, tuck your shirt under your left armpit and keep it snug against your chest as you swing back. This will prevent your left arm from separating from your body, a common fault with big-chested players. The more connection there is, the easier it is to keep the club swinging on the correct path, so you can transfer maximum power to the ball.

A good way to feel how much hip rotation is needed in the backswing is to try this drill made famous by fellow endomorph Julius Boros. Take your address position with a driver and swing the club back to hip height with your right arm only, extending your arm as far as you can. Next, reach over with your left hand and place it on the grip. You probably can't do it at first because your chest, or tummy, gets in the way. The only way to join your left hand to the grip is to rotate your right hip straight back. Perform this drill several times to create a more efficient backswing turn and more width, which, when combined with your strength, should have you hitting balls toward the moon.

SUMMARY: YOUR BODY (TYPE) TELLS ALL

Your body type in large part determines the size and shape of your swing, as well as how much flexibility you have—and where you need to focus your attention when strengthening and conditioning your golf-specific muscles. For example, a taller, slender golfer has plenty of flexibility but little muscle, and he therefore needs to focus more on Series B and C (Chapters Thirteen and Fourteen) and those exercises that will add more strength and endurance to his core. A stocky golfer, however, has too much bulk and not enough flexibility, and should pay close attention to Series A (Chapter Twelve) and those exercises that will add more elasticity to his muscles and increase his range of motion.

Your body type is also a good indicator of what type of injuries you're prone to suffer. Know what the advantages and disadvantages are to being tall, stocky, or athletic, and use that knowledge to minimize those disadvantages to become the golfer you want to become.

HYBRID PLAYERS

The leverage, arc, and width designations are only starting points, says Adams. "Just about every player is a hybrid of two or all three of these types," says Adams. "What you have to do is find out which one you most closely resemble."

If it's power you seek, it's good to be a leverage player with some arc characteristics, says Adams. Tiger Woods fits this mold, as does Ernie Els. Michelle Wie and Vijay Singh, both very tall, powerful hitters, are more arc players with leverage. Appearance-wise, John Daly looks as though he's all width, but he's actually a combo of arc and width because of the tremendous distance his clubhead travels during the swing.

CHAPTER NINE

THE MENTAL GAME: WHAT TO DO WHEN THE WHEELS FALL OFF

You're cruising along for six holes when suddenly you duck-hook your tee shot into the adjacent fairway on the next hole. After punching out, you push your approach shot fifty yards to the right of the green, then follow that by burying your pitch into a deep greenside bunker. Three shots later, you walk away with a triple-bogey 7, ready to implode on the next tee. Appalled with your performance on the previous hole, you pop up your next tee shot. For the next several holes, you struggle to regain any kind of consistency in your game, growing increasingly more frustrated with each and every shot.

Sound familiar? It might. Whether you're a 5-handicapper, a 15, or a 25, you're sure to hit rough patches every now and then. Some golfers can't go eighteen holes without fumbling the ball around for several holes. The wheels fall off and they're left scrambling to put them back on. Yet somehow, great players find a way to bounce back. They have their bad days, sure, but rarely do they let them get out of control. They manage to get it "in the house" with a respectable score, even if they don't have their "A" game, as Tiger Woods would say, or even their "B" or "C" game.

How do they turn a 78 into a 72? According to golf coaches Pia Nilsson and Lynn Marriott, coauthors of the book *Every Shot Must Have a Purpose*, it's that they're able to recognize the trouble signs and take action before it gets out of hand. They're also very aware of their tendencies and mannerisms when they're playing well, so when the first signs of the wheels falling off present themselves, they can apply this knowledge to their game.

In this chapter, you'll find several strategies designed to help you "stop the bleeding." Nobody is perfect, especially over eighteen holes of golf. You're going to hit your fair share of bad shots and wonder why it is you ever woke up at five A.M. to play this morning. How you deal with these errors might mean the difference between posting a good score or a forgettable one.

PROCESS VERSUS OUTCOME

When things go bad, most golfers start to project ahead. They lose sight of the process, or the current shot at hand, and instead focus on the outcome (i.e., "What if I slice this ball into the trees? If I hit it into the bunker here, I'll be lucky to make double bogey"). In most instances, the outcome is a negative image or thought. You start to believe something that hasn't happened yet. "You have to stop the movie, stop projecting ahead, and get your mind back into the present," says Marriott.

One way to stop fast-forwarding is to become more engrossed in the process itself, says Jonathan Katz, a clinical sports psychologist based in New York. "The advantage to playing golf is that after you hit a shot, you have time to evaluate it as you walk to your next shot," says Katz. "But you have to assess it quickly, and then move on to the next shot. As you approach the ball, you need to be thinking, 'OK, I'm behind this tree, now how do I get myself out of this?' You can't be thinking, 'Oh God, I missed another fairway,' or 'Why did the ball have to land behind this tree?' It's no longer about being in the fairway, it's about advancing the ball from out behind the tree as close to the green as possible."

Analyze, don't criticize. If you follow through with a good process, the outcome generally takes care of itself. If you hit the ball solid off the tee but it leaks out into the right rough, focus on the fact that you made good contact, but also consider what you did to turn it into something of a negative shot. Look at it in a constructive way, analyze it, and then move on.

It also helps to be aware of your tendencies, both emotionally and physically, when things start to unravel. This way, you can catch them before they get the better of you, and then do something about them. Some of these warning signs include tight facial and upper-body muscles (you can't make a complete shoulder turn); quick, darting eyes (your eyes no longer gaze at the target, they just glance at it); and increased self-criticism, rapid breathing, and faster body movements (golfers tend to pick up the pace when they're struggling). "If you sense your tempo is getting too quick, try using a verbal cue or visual image to slow you down," says Nilsson. "Maybe you say, 'One aaannndd two,' or visualize a calm sea at the top of your swing."

Creating a physical diversion, such as bouncing in place or wagging your tongue, can also help to relieve the stress associated with the outcome of a particular shot. Games also serve as a good distraction. Nilsson, the former coach of the Swedish National Team, would have her players participate in a game that awarded one point for every fairway and green hit, one point for every up and down and par, and two points for birdie. The purpose was to get each player to realize that every shot is important.

QUIET THE SELF-CHATTER

When you get nervous, the internal conversation you have with yourself tends to get louder, faster, and more negative. You need to find a way to diffuse the derisive chatter, or what Marriott refers to as "roof brain" chatter. Again, create a diversion that will make this chatter disappear. Hum a tune, sing a song, look up at the trees, or converse with your playing partners—anything to help shift your focus back to the task at hand. Develop your own mantra, as Annika Sorenstam did in winning the second of her back-to-back U.S. Women's Open titles in 1996. Holding a three-shot lead heading into the final round, Sorenstam repeated the words "fairway-green, fairway-green" over and over to herself. It was quite effective—Sorenstam fired a 4-under-par 66 to win going away.

Sorenstam is the only female player to shoot a 59 in LPGA competition. On the men's PGA Tour, David Duval, Chip Beck, and Al Geiberger have all accomplished the feat. What these players will tell you, as will any athlete who's ever been "in the zone," is just how quiet and easy things are when you're hitting perfect shot after perfect shot, or making jump shots from everywhere on the basketball floor. Things slow down, and the internal talk is nearly silenced.

So when things get loud, really loud, reach for the mute button. Step away and go through your preshot routine again, or just wait until the derisive talk goes quiet.

"When a person is stressed, there is a voice inside of them doing the talking," says Nilsson. "The specific distinctions of this voice are what let the body and brain know that it is time to be stressed. Practice changing the tempo, tone, and volume of this internal voice. Recall a voice—perhaps it's your favorite actor's voice—and mimic that voice as you're talking to yourself. The pace, cadence, and volume of the voice is key—as your voice changes, so does your emotional state."

The voice inside your head can be more than just a negative thought, or the fear of missing, says Katz. It can also be a swing thought; anything that gets in the way of you hitting the shot in front of you.

"When you're done playing the round, that's the time to become a little more self-critical and evaluative, not in-between shots," says Katz. "Take stock of what you did well or didn't, but only to assess it and try to correct it. Your overall self-evaluation of your round comes afterward, not in the middle of the game. There's not enough time and energy for that; you need energy to focus on each shot."

"THINK," AND THEN "DO"

One of the most effective ways to focus on the present is to develop a preshot routine. You won't find many tour players walking straight up to their ball, picking a target, and then firing away. They all have a set routine they follow, one that usually starts from behind the ball and takes twenty to thirty seconds to complete. The routine is the same for every full swing shot and helps get them in the correct frame of mind (i.e., in the present) to execute the shot they want to play.

"Your routine should be very familiar to you, and, as such, will provide comfort in times when you're extra nervous or pumped up," says Nilsson.

Marriott and Nilsson advocate that you do all of your thinking behind the ball, in what they refer to as the "Think Box" (*below*). This is where all of your decisions are to be made. It's where you gather information about the shot (How's my lie?

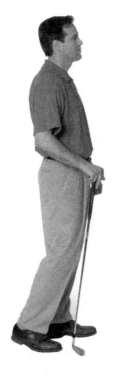

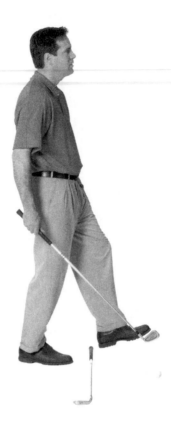

Which direction is the wind blowing and how hard? How far is it to the fairway bunker on the left?). Once you determine the type of shot you want to play, you verbalize it ("I'm going to start the ball at the right edge of the bunker and fade it back toward the center of the fairway") and then visualize it as well.

Approximately midway between the "Think Box" and your ball is the "Decision Line." Once you cross this line (*above*), the cognitive phase stops and you're in what Marriott and Nilsson refer to as the "Do Box." There's no more thinking or evaluating to be done. You've already made your decision and now all that's left to do is connect to your target and execute the game plan.

Most poor shots result from indecisiveness. You'll find many golfers still processing information over the ball when they should be engaged with the target. ("Is this the right club?" "Do I really want to hit it toward the right edge of that bunker?"

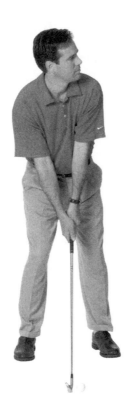

"What did my instructor say about turning my hips out of the way?") Indecision doesn't build confidence, and it sure doesn't produce quality shots. The whole purpose of the preshot routine is to gather information and devise a strategy that gives you the best opportunity to execute the shot at hand. Once you devise a plan, stick to it. Stay committed to your shot. Once you're over the ball, take a slow glance or two at the target (*above*) and then fire away.

BREATHE DEEP

Whenever you are confronted with a stressful situation, such as a forced carry over water or a slick, three-foot putt for par, it helps to slow your breathing. An increase in stress heightens anxiety, which in turn leads to an increase in your serum cortisol

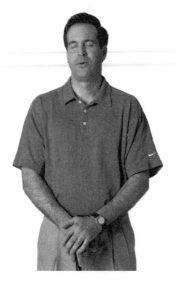

levels (cortisol is a steroid hormone released from the adrenal gland). When these levels get too high, your breathing becomes very rapid and shallow. The muscles in your face and throughout your body begin to tense up, which makes it very difficult to perform your best under pressure.

As you address the ball, take several deep breaths in through your nose and out through your mouth. Imagine that your stomach is a balloon and you're filling it with oxygen as you breathe in. (Your ribs should expand out to your sides.) As you breathe in and out, close your eyes and picture a clear, blue sky. No clouds, no sound, nothing. Inhale to a count of three, then exhale and take another deep breath.

Take two or three deep breaths before starting the club back. By returning to a more natural breathing pattern, you recruit oxygen to your muscles, reducing cortisone levels. You'll relax your grip and get a better feel for the clubhead, which will free up your swing on the golf course.

GO WITH YOUR SECOND SERVE

If you're struggling with your swing and confidence, take a more cautious approach with your game. Don't go into full attack mode, firing at tucked pins or going for every par-5 in two. Take into consideration how you're playing, and then ask yourself, "How many times out of ten can I reasonably pull this shot off?" If it's 50 percent or less, don't make matters worse by being a hero. Settle down and be more realistic. If you can string a few decent holes together in a row, you'll be right back on track.

Dr. Richard Coop, Professor of Educational Psychology at the University of North Carolina at Chapel Hill and a regular contributor to *GOLF Magazine*, suggests taking a "second-serve approach" when coming off a bad hole.

"When tennis players fault on their first serve, they hit a more conservative second serve to better their chances of getting the ball in," Coop wrote in *GOLF Magazine*. "Consider developing a similar technique for tee shots after disastrous holes. Grip down on the driver an inch, maybe even go to a fairway wood, and try to make a smooth, three-quarter swing that advances the ball down the middle with minimal risk."

It's also good to reach for the video replay button, says Coop, especially when your confidence is in dire need of a boost.

"Recall good tee shots you've hit on the hole you're about to play," says Coop. "Or, if you're on an unfamiliar course, try to equate it to a similar tee shot with which you've had success. Always watch your good shots—burn them into your memory—so you can think back on them when you need a psychological boost."

HOW TO NOT BLOW A GASKET

The last thing you want to do is throw a tantrum on the course. For one, you'll embarrass yourself, and two, you might disturb the concentration of one or more of your fellow playing partners. And you certainly don't want to break a club. Bad shots will happen, just as surely as it will rain in Seattle sometime in the next thirty days. You can choose to accept them as part of the game, or you can get all bent out of shape. Beating yourself up over a mistake is a total waste of your time and energy.

The next time you get the urge to bash yourself or throw a club, try the following tricks to keep cool.

Keep Your Head Up

When people get angry and frustrated, or they sulk, they tend to do so with their heads down. Think about it: How many times do you express anguish with your eyes looking up at the sky? Probably never. You express your disgust in a more introverted manner, so it's less visible to the outside. So the next time you hit a poor shot and think of cursing yourself out, look up, not down. Keep your eyes even with or above the horizon. "By raising your head, you become more visually aware of your surroundings," says Marriott. "Your mind sees what your eyes see, providing a distraction from the feelings of anger you are experiencing."

Take a Five-Count

As soon as you know your shot is headed for disaster, start counting very slowly to yourself—one-thousand-one, one-thousand-two, one-thousand-three, etc.—all the way to five. You'll delay your normal response—generally, an instantaneous display of anger—just long enough to prevent it from happening.

Once you're done counting, you need to disassociate yourself from the bad outcome.

"If you hit your tee shot out of bounds, take a few seconds to replay the shot with the desired outcome in mind," says Marriott. "Imagine the ball splitting the fairway; anything to replace the feelings of anger and disappointment usually associated with a bad shot."

Call a Mental Time-Out

You see it in other sports, such as basketball: A team is victimized by a 12–0 run, and the coach calls time-out to allow his players time to regroup and perhaps thwart the other team's momentum. Try doing the same after a particularly bad hole. Talk to one of your playing partners about a movie you recently saw, pull that energy bar you've been saving out of your bag and eat it slowly, or perform one of the eighteen stretches from Chapter Six. By taking your mind off the last hole and putting your attention elsewhere, you should be mentally recharged to play the next shot.

CHAPTER TEN

BONUS ROUND: TIPS ON NUTRITION, HYDRATION, AND MASSAGE

Hall of Fame golf instructor Jim Flick says that golf is "90 percent mental." And the other 10 percent?

"The other 10 percent is mental, too," he says.

Few sports require that you use your brain as much as golf. Consider how much thought goes into your average approach shot—you have to factor in the wind, the pin position, the firmness of the green, the slope of the green, your lie (how the ball is sitting), where the trouble is, how you're swinging the club that day, etc. You might have to contend with past failures on the same hole (e.g., the very last time you were here, you hit the ball in the water and made triple bogey), or you might be coming off a horrendous bogey on the previous hole. Maybe you're headed toward a career-best round and you're trying not to get too far ahead of yourself, or there are some low branches just off the fairway and you're concerned about hitting those. There are so many elements you have to manage during the course of eighteen holes—not just strategically, but emotionally, too—that you're going to need all of the brain energy you can muster.

In order to maintain focus for four-plus hours, it's important to eat and hydrate correctly before, during, and after the round. This doesn't mean you should stop at the snack hut after the 9th hole and order a hot dog and a Coke. When you schedule a round of golf, you should be thinking about what to eat and drink before you tee off, and what to take with you out on the course. You should be as concerned about nutrition as you are about your flying right elbow or occasional duck-hook. Keep your mind sharp, and your game will follow.

BOTTOMS UP: REPLACING LOST FLUIDS

Water can be hazardous on the course, but it can also wreak havoc with your performance if you don't take in enough of it before and during play. This also includes sports drinks such as Gatorade, which provide essential carbohydrates and electrolytes, including sodium. Most people walk or run around dehydrated because they underestimate just how much sweat they lose during exercise. It's not entirely our fault—our bodies often do a poor job of telling us when we are dehydrated—but it is recommended that you replace 100 percent of the sweat you lose during exercise.

As you exercise, your body temperature naturally rises. You release sweat as a way of keeping your body cool. How much fluid you drink depends on how much sweat you lose. A good rule of thumb is typically four to six ounces of water every fifteen to twenty minutes, says Heidi Skolnik, a sports nutrition consultant for the New York Giants football team and the School of American Ballet. If you want to be absolutely sure, weigh yourself before and after play on a typical warm summer day and see how much water weight you lose. Then add back in the amount of water you ingested during the round to determine your average sweat rate. For example, if you weighed 220 pounds before you teed off and 216 afterward, then you lost approximately four pounds of water weight, a sweat loss of sixty-four ounces. But if you drank two twelve-ounce bottles of water during the course of play, you must figure this amount in, which brings your total sweat loss to eighty-eight ounces. You divide up eighty-eight ounces over four hours, and it comes to roughly twenty-two ounces of sweat per hour. You would need to drink 5.5 ounces of water or sports drink every fifteen minutes to be properly hydrated.

The hotter the conditions, the more sweat you must replace. Failure to drink enough water in these conditions can lead to a loss of concentration, fatigue, muscle tightness, and, in the worst cases, heatstroke. The latter tends to happen more frequently in dry heat conditions where golfers are more susceptible to dehydration. This is because in dry heat (which you'll find in Las Vegas, Palm Springs, and the Arizona desert), there's little to no moisture in the air, so your perspiration evaporates

TO DETERMINE YOUR SWEAT RATE:

1. On a typically hot summer day, weigh yourself prior to the start of your round. Example: 200 lbs.
2. Weigh yourself after the round is complete. Example: 197 lbs.
3. Subtract line two (197 lbs.) from line one (200 lbs.) to determine how much water weight you lost. Example: 200−197=3 lbs., which is the equivalent of forty-eight ounces of water.
4. Add back how much water you drank during the course of play. Example: You drank two sixteen-ounce bottles of water, or thirty-two ounces.
5. Add to the original weight lost to figure your total sweat loss. Example: 48+32=80 ounces.
6. Divide by the total time spent on the course (in hours) to figure out your sweat rate. Example: $\frac{80}{4}$ (hours)=20 ounces per hour, or five ounces every fifteen minutes.

You should make sure to drink twenty ounces of water every hour.

much more quickly on your skin. As a result, it's harder to recognize just how much you're sweating. You don't feel as hot as you would in humid conditions because the sweat is leaving your body, not sticking to it. This can be very dangerous, because while you might not be feeling the heat as much, your body is still pumping out a ton of water. Don't take any chances. Force yourself to ingest just as much water as you would under humid conditions—drink at least six ounces of water before you tee off on every hole.

GATORADE VS. COFFEE

The old Gatorade commercials encouraged viewers to "Be like Mike," as in NBA great Michael Jordan, who frequently could be seen endorsing his favorite orange-colored drink. Sports drinks have become increasingly popular over the last ten years, and with good reason. Products such as Gatorade, POWERade, and Amino Vital are excellent choices during exercise because they contain carbohydrates and important electrolytes such as sodium and potassium. Carbohydrates provide energy to your working muscles so you're just as strong on the 18th hole as you were on the 2nd hole. Electrolytes help your body distribute water (i.e., sweat), which is why your skin often looks like the outside of a salted pretzel after an intense workout.

Perhaps the greatest benefit to sports drinks such as Gatorade is that they taste good. They encourage you to drink more, so you're more likely to rehydrate yourself and less likely to become dehydrated during the course of exercising.

Caffeinated beverages such as coffee and soda are okay, as long as you take in other fluids along the way such as water and Gatorade. Neither coffee nor Coke is a hydrator, so they won't prevent you from becoming dehydrated. Coffee is also a stimulant, so pay careful attention to how your body reacts on the tee or over a putt after you've had a cup of java. Some people are very sensitive to coffee. If you have too much adrenaline or your stroke is jerky, you may want to back off the coffee and stick with water or juice as your beverage of choice in the morning.

As for alcohol, it should be avoided until after the round, especially in warm and humid conditions where you're prone to sweat a lot more. Alcohol will not only impair your performance by limiting your endurance, coordination, and concentration, but it will also dehydrate you. Alcohol is a diuretic and stimulates fluid loss, which is something you don't want when you're losing a lot of sweat in the first place.

EAT FOR BETTER STAMINA

While golf doesn't have the same cardiovascular strains as other sports, such as tennis, basketball, or soccer, it does require more stamina because you're out there on the playing field much longer. An average round of golf takes roughly four to five hours to complete, so if you want to sustain your energy and strength for a full eighteen holes, you have to eat properly. What and how often you eat will affect your ability to focus, your timing, and your hand-eye coordination. If you're running low on carbohydrates, and your blood sugar level is dropping, it's going to be extremely difficult to perform up to your expectations.

The recommended daily caloric intake for physically active men is 2,700 calories (2,000 for women), according to the National Academy of Sciences. This means that if you have a seven A.M. tee time, by noon you should have consumed roughly 1,300 calories, says Heidi Skolnik. If you go out there and all you have for breakfast is a piece of toast or a Nutri-Grain bar, you're already at a huge deficit come midday.

Skolnik suggests you consume about 500 to 700 calories before teeing off. Good breakfast choices include whole grains (oatmeal, bagel, toast), protein and dairy products (skim milk, yogurt, eggs, peanut butter, nuts), and fruits (bananas, grapefruit, orange juice). On the course, Skolnik recommends munching on some form of trail mix (with Cheerios, pumpkin seeds, or pretzel sticks), an energy bar or banana, dried fruit or cereal, and nuts (especially almonds). "You want things that are easily tolerated by your system and easy to get down," says Skolnik. "Keep your meal on the lighter side (e.g., eat half a deli sandwich versus a hoagie) and stay away from fried foods, such as french fries and fish sticks."

On the evening before a big tournament or match, make sure to eat a well-rounded meal. A quarter of your plate should come from proteins and the rest from grain, starch, fruit, and vegetables, which are all loaded with carbohydrates. Again, don't overindulge in alcohol, because it's dehydrating. Save it for after the big round when you're celebrating the slew of birdies you just made.

Also make sure to get a good night's rest (at least eight hours) the day before the start of the tournament, when you don't have to get up so early and you won't be as anxious.

TIPS TO BEAT THE HEAT

Since golf is predominantly a summertime activity, it's important that you know what to do when the thermometer is rising higher than a Phil Mickelson flop shot. Monitor the weather forecast during the week. If the forecast calls for hazy, hot, and humid conditions over the weekend or on the day you're scheduled to play, consider hitting the water bottle early. Start hydrating yourself forty-eight hours before your round by drinking extra water—at least two thirty-two-ounce bottles—each day. Protect yourself from the sun's rays as well, covering your head with a wide-brimmed hat (e.g., a straw hat) that keeps the sun off your neck and ears. If you don't have such a hat, consider pulling up the collar on your shirt so it covers the back of your neck.

Here are some other ways to keep cool:

- Find shade wherever you can. If trees are sparse, consider bringing an umbrella to shade yourself from the sun.
- Stick a small hand towel in a cooler of ice water, or ask a cart person to keep one cool for you. When you get a break in the action, take the towel

out and drape it over the back of your neck, or rub it across your forehead.

- Wear light-colored, breathable clothing, including socks. Stay away from dark colors such as black, navy blue, and red, because they absorb heat more readily and raise your body temperature.

- Chill out, literally. Take it slow, and try and keep your temper tantrums to a minimum. You don't want to become increasingly agitated in conditions that are suited to overheating.

RUB IT IN, RUB IT IN

From time to time, your hamstrings, back muscles, hip flexors, shoulders, and other golf-specific muscles will feel sore from overuse or general stiffness. In these instances, when you feel more like the Tin Man than Tiger Woods, you might want to consider some form of massage therapy. In conjunction with stretching and cardiovascular exercise, a good massage will enhance your flexibility and range of motion, as well as increase circulation (i.e., blood flow) to these muscles. More significantly, it flushes out the toxins, lactic acid, and other forms of gunk that build up in your muscles after heavy usage. When not expelled, these by-products stick around like plaque and cause your muscles to ache.

The two most common forms of massage therapy are deep- and soft-tissue massage. Deep-tissue therapy is just that—a penetrating type of massage that works the deep connective tissue surrounding your muscles, tendons, and joints and the skeletal muscles close to the bone. The massage therapist applies firm, constant pressure with his elbows, thumbs, fists, and forearms to push deep into the muscle and connective tissue, pulling it from end to end. "You gradually apply pressure to the area until you feel the tissue release," says Sandra Hewick, a licensed massage therapist based in San Diego. "You feel the muscle drop. It's like peeling through an onion— you have to sink into it and it will release."

Deep-tissue massage helps break up lesions, scar tissue, and other toxins that can form when the muscle becomes inflamed. There is generally some soreness after treatment, so make sure to have this type of massage after you've finished playing, not before.

Soft-tissue massage is gentler and more relaxing than deep-tissue work and safe to have before and after golf. This Swedish style of massage employs longer, more sweeping strokes with the fingertips or palms. It helps stimulate blood flow to the muscles, bringing nutrients to the muscles to help flush them out so there's no delayed onset of muscle soreness. It helps to keep the muscle long and pliable.

"Golfers are generally very tight in the front of the chest and in the mid-back region, around the thoracic spine," says Lisa Fierstein, a licensed massage therapist and physical therapist also based in San Diego. "I tend to do a lot of work in these areas because they're constantly being pulled forward in people's everyday lives. Effective massage treatments can help balance you out."

Fierstein also recommends using a foam roller to open up the mid-back region and undo the forward bend created by desk-job syndrome. Lie on the floor with your knees bent, feet on the floor, and arms out to your sides. Position the foam roller underneath (parallel to) your spine, with your head supported by the roller. Lie there for several minutes, moving your arms up and down along the ground as though you were making a snow angel. "This will make your posture more upright," says Fierstein, "and create the extension you need for golf."

PART TWO

GOLF Rx SERIES
A, B, AND C

CHAPTER ELEVEN

CONDITIONING YOUR CORE:
AN INTRODUCTION TO
GOLF RX SERIES A, B, AND C

No sport is associated more with lower-back pain than golf. What the throwing shoulder and elbow is to a baseball pitcher, the lower back is to a golfer. The twisting motion of the swing combined with the sudden acceleration and deceleration forces being applied to the lower back make it an easy target for discomfort and injury. Keeping it strong and flexible, along with the core muscles that support it, is not only essential to playing regularly, but is a must if you want to swing better and lower your scores.

In 2001, I led a study on the prevalence of lower-back pain in professional golfers at the PGA Tour's Buick Classic in Westchester County, New York. Forty-two golfers (mean age of thirty-one) were tested, one-third of whom had experienced lower-back pain for a period of at least two weeks in the previous twelve months. The remaining two-thirds had no such prior history.

Using a goniometer device to detail range of motion, we ran a number of different tests on each golfer, measuring, among other things, the internal rotation of the lead and non-lead hips, and the flexion (bending forward) and extension of the lumbar spine. What we found among the symptomatic golfers was a high correlation between the loss of internal rotation in the lead hip and decreased lumbar extension—the process of bending backward—and lower-back pain. A lack of hip mobility put too much load on the lumbar spine, contributing to the lower-back pain. Those golfers with healthy backs did not have a significant decrease in the internal and external rotation of the lead hip.

Out of this research was born *Back Rx* (2004, Gotham Books), a yoga- and Pilates-based program designed to restore flexibility and prevent future injuries to the lower back. But being a former professional tennis player myself, I wanted to take it one step further for golfers and design a program that would not only prevent injuries but enhance performance, so that you could hit the ball longer and more consistently than ever before. This is the goal of *Golf Rx* and the exercises that follow in Series A, B, and C: to not only improve your back health so you can enjoy the game for a lifetime, but also to revitalize your swing so you can play your best golf in the near future.

Golf Rx is a golf-specific conditioning program designed to increase your range of motion and the efficiency of your swing so you can hit the ball more precisely, with more clubhead speed and power. By golf-specific, I mean core-specific. You rely almost exclusively on your body's midsection to supply maximum force to the golf ball. More importantly, it is the core's job to dissipate this energy so that the lower back doesn't take on too much stress. Golf-specific training conditions the muscles of your core for very short, quick bursts of activity, which you must perform repeatedly over the course of four-plus hours in golf. Whereas with a marathon you condition your body for one long, constant burst of energy over several hours, in golf-specific training you condition your core for sporadic bursts of acceleration and deceleration that you must perform in a controlled manner.

Golf Rx is the perfect off-season exercise program because it not only restores flexibility to the muscles that need it most, it builds strength and stamina in the core so that your body is able to withstand the rigors of a full golf season. I see many more golf-related back injuries in the spring than at any other time of year because the core is not yet conditioned to fire and brake so frequently. The core is deconditioned and fatigued, and you need to build up more endurance in it before you resume a full playing schedule.

Series C emphasizes endurance, while Series A and B focus on developing flexibility and strength in the core. Each series should be performed a minimum of three times per week, up to five times per week, and should take no more than fifteen to twenty minutes to complete. There are no weights, cords, golf clubs, or training aids needed to perform the exercises; all you need is an exercise mat and some comfortable clothes. Make sure your muscles are warmed up before you start (a hot shower works just as well as riding a stationary bike for a few minutes), and remember to take slow, sustained breaths as you perform each exercise.

Most importantly, do not start the exercises in *Golf Rx* Series A, B, and C if you are currently suffering from knee or back pain. If the pain has been present for more than one week, see a doctor.

I recommend everyone start with Series A and progress from there, but if you're fairly flexible and in good condition you might want to jump right into Series B. It all depends on your level of fitness. The exercises get increasingly difficult from Series A to Series C, but the basic principles remain the same: 1) Improve your general fitness; and 2) condition your golf-specific core muscles so you can play your best golf, injury-free.

Here is a short breakdown of each series.

SERIES A: CORE FLEXIBILITY

Before you can build the second floor or the top floor, you need a solid foundation. This is what *Golf Rx* Series A provides. The fifteen exercises in Series A will improve your flexibility and range of motion so that you're able to perform a basic golf swing without too many physical restrictions. Increased core flexibility is at the heart of *Golf Rx*, which is why I recommend everyone start with Series A before attempting Series B or C. Beginners and seniors should definitely begin with Series A, and, in most cases, seniors shouldn't advance beyond Series A. With better core flexibility and more mobility in their joints, seniors should see a big improvement in their distance off the tee and their performance after just a few weeks of starting Series A.

SERIES B: CORE STRENGTH

Much like today's fast-food choices, the game of golf has been super-sized over the last twenty years. Courses are getting longer, clubheads are getting bigger, and the ball is flying higher and farther than ever before. It's become very much a power game, even on the amateur level, and to keep up you have to be stronger and fitter than ever. This is where *Golf Rx* Series B comes in. Series B forces you to hold each stretch longer than Series A, challenging your core muscles to work harder to keep your body stable and thus increasing your core strength. Combined with good swing mechanics, Series B will provide you with the tools necessary to add ten more yards to your tee shots.

SERIES C: CORE ENDURANCE

Between your warm-up, practice swings, and actual swings, you're asking your body to swing well in excess of a hundred times during the course of a typical round of golf. That's expending a lot of energy. Series C increases the number of repetitions per exercise and makes your core work for longer stretches of time, building endurance in these muscles so your swing can hold up for eighteen holes. Series C trains your core to fire again and again at a high rate of speed, so your swing is as powerful on the 18th hole as it is on the first hole. It prevents your core from fatiguing, one of the major contributors to injuries—specifically, back and hip injuries—in golfers.

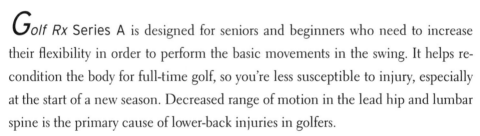

CHAPTER TWELVE

REGAINING SOME FLEXIBILITY: *GOLF Rx* SERIES A

Golf Rx Series A is designed for seniors and beginners who need to increase their flexibility in order to perform the basic movements in the swing. It helps recondition the body for full-time golf, so you're less susceptible to injury, especially at the start of a new season. Decreased range of motion in the lead hip and lumbar spine is the primary cause of lower-back injuries in golfers.

Perform the following series of exercises three times a week, holding each stretch for a count of five deep breaths in and out.

KNEE TO CHEST WITH WRIST STRETCH

- Lie flat on your back with your arms straight at your sides and knees bent, feet flat on the floor.

- Loop your right arm under the crook of your right knee (right palm pointing outward), and slowly bring your knee toward your chest until your thigh is perpendicular to the floor. Your shin should be parallel to the floor and your toes pointed upward. Raise your shoulders just off the floor to open up your hip flexors, located deep in your thighs.

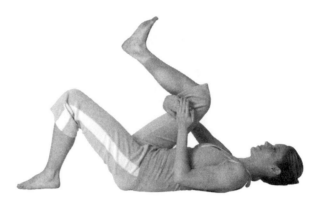

- At the end of the stretch, gently push the fingers of your right hand back toward your right leg using the fingers of your left hand. You should feel a good stretch on the underside of your right forearm.
- Hold this position for a count of five deep breaths in and out, and then return to the starting position.
- Repeat with the opposite leg, bringing your left knee toward your chest while stretching out the wrist flexors on the underside of your left forearm. You'll also feel a gentle stretch in your hip flexors and lower back, increasing the range of motion in your trunk.

ILIOTIBIAL BAND STRETCH

- Lie flat on your back with your legs straight and arms extended out to the sides, forming a "T."
- Raise your right leg several inches off the floor and cross it over your left leg, allowing it to fall toward your left hip. Make sure your toes are pointed upward and your right leg is straight.
- Hold for a count of five deep breaths in and out.
- Return to the starting position and repeat with the other leg.

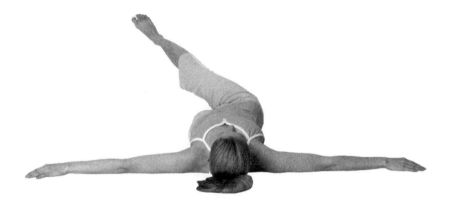

This exercise stretches the outside of your hip, the iliotibial band, and your buttocks, increasing the range of motion in your hips so you can make a better turn back and through.

- Lie flat on your back with your legs bent and arms extended out to the sides, forming a "T."
- Cross your left leg over your bent right knee so that it's in contact with the outside of your knee.
- Use the weight of your left leg to apply pressure to the outside of your right knee, bringing it toward your left hip.
- Hold the stretch for at least five deep breaths in and out, then return to the starting position, with both knees bent.

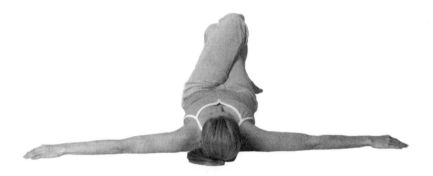

- Repeat with the opposite leg to help increase the internal rotation of your hips, which is pivotal in reducing the load on your back in the follow-through.

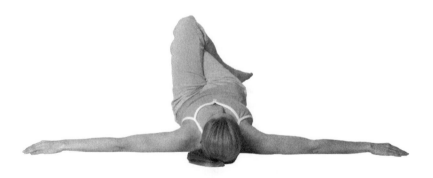

ABDOMINAL CRUNCH

- Lie on your back with your hands behind your head. Slowly raise one knee at a time into a bent position, so that both feet are flat on the floor.

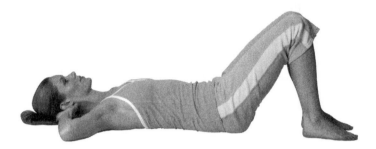

- Tuck your chin into your chest and slowly raise your shoulders so the tips of your shoulder blades are off the floor. The bottoms of your shoulder blades should remain on the floor.
- Look at your navel as you curl your head and shoulders up toward the ceiling, drawing your abs in toward your spine for additional support. Make sure to keep your ears in line with your shoulders.

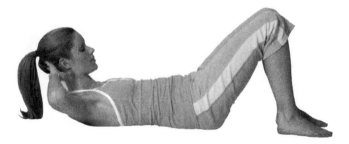

- Hold for a count of five deep breaths in and out and exhale as you bring your head back to the floor.

This exercise targets your upper abdominal muscles, which are extremely important in maintaining your posture throughout the golf swing.

- Lie flat on your back with your left leg straight and right foot touching the inside of your left knee, forming a figure four with your lower body. Look straight up at the sky and imagine the line between your neck and spine lengthening.
- Reach across your chest with your left arm, and gently pull your right elbow even farther across your body with the back of your left hand. At the same time, try to get the outside of your right knee close to the floor.
- Hold for a count of five deep breaths in and out, then repeat with the opposite leg and arm.

This exercise stretches the posterior capsules at the back of each shoulder, improving your overall posture and your ability to make a full shoulder turn. It also increases external rotation in the hips.

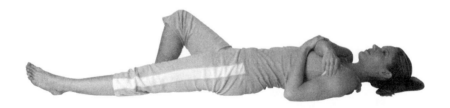

LUMBAR ROTATION DOUBLE KNEE

- Lie flat on your back with knees bent, feet flat on the floor, and both arms extended out to the side with your palms facing the ceiling.
- Slowly lower your knees to one side (feet and knees together) as far as you comfortably can, keeping your shoulders flat on the floor.
- Turn your head in the opposite direction of where your knees are going. Hold for a count of five deep breaths in and out, and repeat the stretch lowering your knees to the other side.

This exercise will improve your spinal rotation, increasing the difference between your shoulder and hip turns on the backswing.

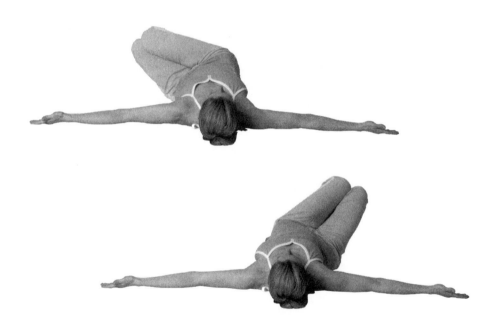

- Lie flat on your back with your arms at your sides. Gently raise your left knee into a bent position while keeping your right leg straight, toes pointing toward the ceiling.
- Slowly raise your right leg off the floor until your right thigh is even with your left thigh. Try to keep your lower back flat on the floor, drawing your abs in toward your spine to help stabilize the spine.

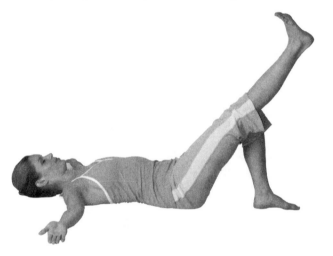

- Hold for a count of five deep breaths, return to the starting position, and then repeat with the opposite leg.

This exercise strengthens your hip flexors, quadriceps, and lower abs, and helps lengthen your hamstrings.

BOUND-ANGLE SEATED STRETCH

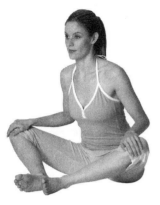

- Take a seated position on the floor with both legs bent. Grasp your ankles and slowly draw one foot at a time in toward your groin so that the heels of your feet are touching, forming a diamond with your lower body.
- Keeping your back straight and your arms and shoulders relaxed, bend forward from your hips as far as your range of motion will allow.
- You should feel a good stretch through your inner-thigh muscles. Hold for a count of five deep breaths in and out.

This exercise stretches your groin and inner-thigh muscles, increasing the range of motion in your hips so you can make a better turn behind the ball.

CROSS-LEGGED SITTING-FORWARD BEND

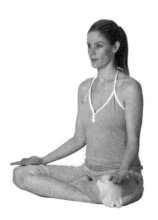

- Sit up on the floor in a simple cross-legged position, ankles touching the floor.
- Extend your arms out in front of you so that the backs of your hands are resting on the insides of your knees, with the palms facing upward.
- Bend slightly forward from your hips, elongating your spine as you press your hands into your knees.

This FABERE (Flexion, ABduction, External Rotation, and Extension) stretch targets just about every muscle in the hip, very important in preventing lower-back injuries.

- Sit up on the floor with your left leg straight and your right knee bent. Cross your right leg over your left so that the outside of your right foot is touching the outside of your left knee.
- Place your right hand on the floor beside you for additional support.
- Grasp the outside of your right knee with your left hand and pull the knee gently toward your left arm.
- Keeping your back as straight as possible, bend forward from your hips— just as though you were sticking your butt out—until you feel a stretch across your right hip and buttocks.
- Hold for a count of five deep breaths in and out and repeat with the opposite leg, stretching your left hip and buttocks.

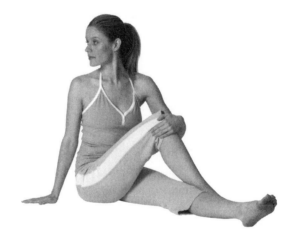

BACK EXTENSION

- Lie on your stomach with your thighs and toes touching the floor, and your elbows tucked under your shoulders, palms flat on the floor.

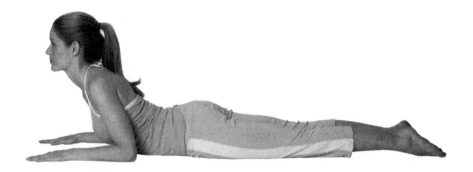

- Lengthen your legs out away from your hips, then slowly press your body backward just enough so your navel clears the floor. Feel as though your shoulder blades are staying down and back as you lift your navel off the floor. Hold the position for five deep breaths in and out.

You should feel a gentle stretch in your lower back, but nothing that should cause any pain. This exercise also works your abdominal muscles.

- Stand up straight with your feet as wide as your shoulder blades and your arms hanging comfortably at your sides. Bring your arms up in front of you and join your hands together as though in prayer.

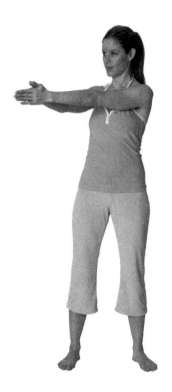 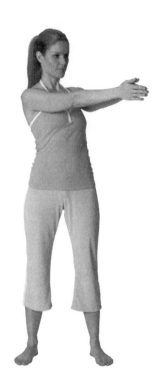

- Slowly turn your upper body to one side. Keep your arms and neck in one continuous straight line as you twist, and turn only as far as your range of motion will allow.
- Hold the position for five deep breaths in and out, then slowly face front and repeat to the other side. You should feel a good stretch in your spine as well as the posterior portions of your shoulders, which will help improve your turn both back and through during each swing.

HIP-ABDUCTOR STRETCH

- Stand straight up with your arms extended diagonally out in front you, at a 45-degree angle, for balance.
- Lift your right leg directly out to the side until you feel a good stretch on the outside of your right thigh. Make sure to line up the center of your forehead, chest, and navel with the inside of your left ankle as you push your leg out. This will prevent you from swaying too much with your lower body.
- Hold the position for a count of five deep breaths in and out. Return your right foot to the starting position and repeat on the opposite leg to strengthen your hip-abductor muscles, which are responsible for moving your legs away from your body.

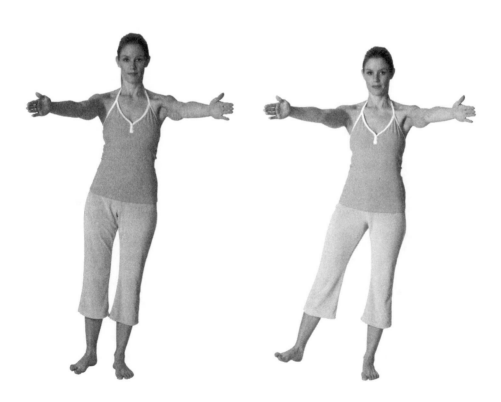

- Stand up straight with your feet shoulder-width apart, knees slightly bent, and arms extended out to your sides, forming a letter "T."
- Slowly twist your upper body to the left as you reach your right hand toward your left foot. It's okay if you don't touch your toes.
- Look back at your left arm as you reach for your left foot, making sure not to lift your head and spine up.
- Hold the position for a count of five deep breaths in and out and return to the starting position. Then reach your left hand toward your right foot.

This exercise will help improve your spinal rotation and increase your hamstring flexibility.

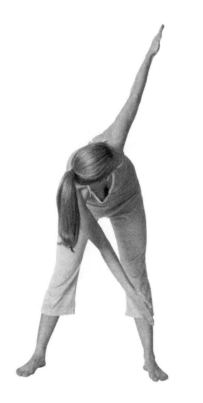 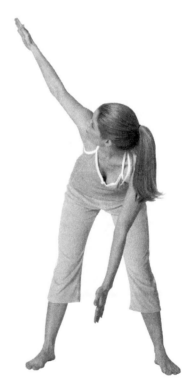

STANDING TREE POSE

- Stand up straight with your arms at your sides and your eyes fixed on a stationary point directly in front of you. Lift your right foot up and place the sole of your foot against the inside of your left ankle. The ball of your right foot should be touching the floor.
- Exhale as you sweep your arms up above your head, gently pressing your right foot into your left ankle as you reach for the sky.
- Hold for a count of five deep breaths in and out, fixing your eyes on a point directly in front of you to help improve your balance. The center of your forehead, chest, and navel should all line up with the inside of your left ankle.

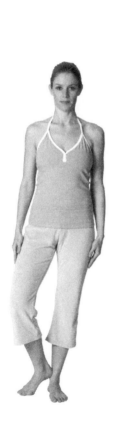
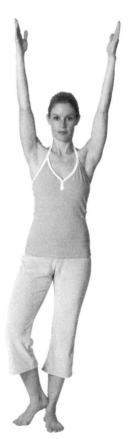

- Return to the starting position and repeat with your left foot joining the inside of your right ankle. This exercise will help improve your balance on the standing leg while also engaging your core muscles for support.

Congratulations! You've now completed *Golf Rx* Series A. To learn how to stretch out your drives, proceed on to *Golf Rx* Series B.

CHAPTER THIRTEEN

ADDING STRENGTH AND DISTANCE:
GOLF Rx SERIES B

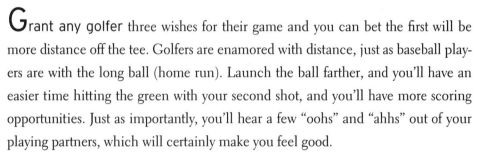

Grant any golfer three wishes for their game and you can bet the first will be more distance off the tee. Golfers are enamored with distance, just as baseball players are with the long ball (home run). Launch the ball farther, and you'll have an easier time hitting the green with your second shot, and you'll have more scoring opportunities. Just as importantly, you'll hear a few "oohs" and "ahhs" out of your playing partners, which will certainly make you feel good.

Golf Rx Series B adds a strength component to Series A by requiring you to hold each stretch longer—seven full breaths instead of five. It helps recruit more of the golf-specific core muscles, since your body weight is providing more resistance with each prolonged stretch.

A more powerful core translates into more yards off the tee. So if you're looking to add ten or more yards to your drives, Series B is for you.

- Lie flat on your back with your arms straight at your sides and your knees bent, feet flat on the floor.
- Loop your right arm under the crook of your right knee and slowly bring your knee toward your right shoulder. Try to get the knee to touch your right shoulder without lifting your shoulders off the floor.

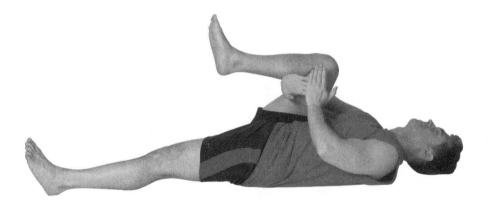

- At the end of the stretch, gently push the fingers of your right hand back toward you using the fingers of your left hand. You should feel a good stretch on the underside of your right forearm.
- Hold this position for a count of seven deep breaths in and out, then return to the starting position.
- Repeat with the opposite leg, bringing your left knee toward your left shoulder while stretching out your left wrist.

ILIOTIBIAL BAND STRETCH

- Lie flat on your back with your legs straight and arms extended out to the sides, forming a "T."
- Raise your right leg several inches off the floor and cross it over your left leg, allowing it to fall toward your left hip. Make sure your toes are pointed straight upward.

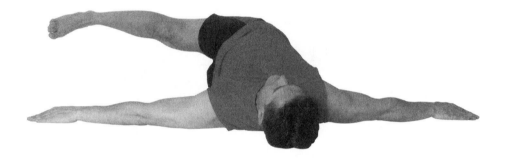

- Try to get your right heel to touch the floor while keeping both shoulders on the floor. Hold this position for a count of seven deep breaths in and out.
- Return to the starting position and repeat with the other leg.

This exercise stretches the outside of each hip, the iliotibial band, and your buttocks, increasing the range of motion in your hips so you can make a better turn back and through.

- Lie flat on your back with your legs bent and arms extended out to the sides, forming a "T."
- Cross your left leg over your bent right knee so that it's in contact with the outside of your knee.

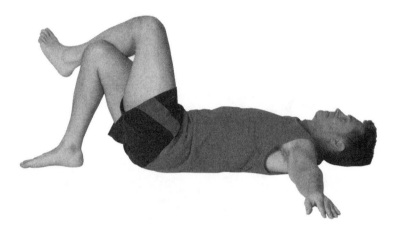

- Use the weight of your left leg to apply pressure to the outside of your right knee, bringing it all the way down to the floor.

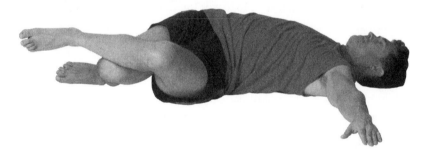

- Hold the stretch for at least seven deep breaths in and out, making sure to keep both shoulders on the floor.
- Repeat with the opposite leg to increase the internal rotation of your hips, which is pivotal to reducing the stress placed on your lower back in the follow-through.

ABDOMINAL CRUNCH

- Lie on your back with your hands behind your head, left knee bent, and right leg straight. Slowly raise your right leg off the floor until it's parallel to your left thigh. Make sure your toes are pointing up toward the ceiling.
- Tuck your chin into your chest and slowly raise your head and shoulders so that your shoulder blades are completely off the floor.
- Look at your navel or hips as you curl your head and shoulders up toward the ceiling, drawing your abs in toward your spine for additional support. Focus on relaxing your head and neck.

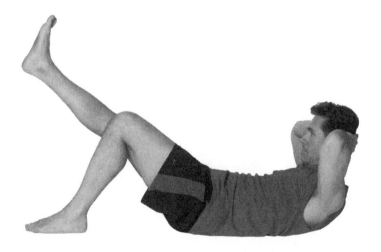

- Hold for a count of seven deep breaths in and out and exhale as you bring your head back to the floor.

Raising your leg off the floor helps strengthen your lower abdominal muscles. This exercise also targets your upper abs, hamstrings, and calves.

- Lie flat on your back with your left leg straight and right knee bent. Cross your bent leg over your left knee, resting the outside of your right foot on top of your thigh, just above the knee.
- Reach across your chest with your left arm, and pull your right elbow even farther across your body with your left hand. Try to get your right index finger to touch the floor just outside of your left shoulder.
- At the same time, try to get the outside of your right knee to touch the floor.
- Hold for a count of seven deep breaths in and out, then repeat with the opposite leg and arm.

This exercise stretches the posterior capsules at the back of each shoulder and also increases external rotation of the hips.

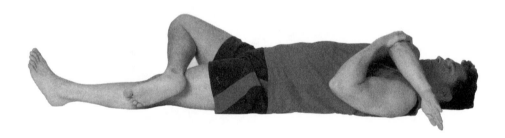

LUMBAR ROTATION DOUBLE KNEE

- Lie flat on your back with your knees bent, feet flat on the floor, and both arms extended out to the side with your palms facing the ceiling.

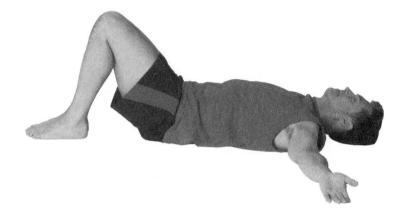

- Slowly lower both knees to one side (feet and knees together) until the bottom knee touches the floor, keeping your shoulders flat on the floor.

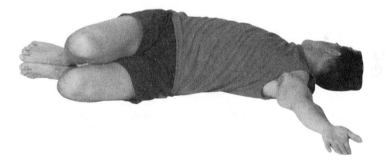

- Turn your head in the opposite direction of where your knees are going. Hold for a count of seven deep breaths in and out, then repeat the stretch, lowering your knees to the other side.

This exercise will improve your spinal rotation, increasing the difference between your shoulder and hip turns on the backswing for a more powerful coil.

- Lie flat on your back with both arms at your sides, left knee bent, and right leg straight on the floor.

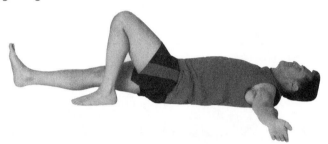

- Raise your right leg up and down—quick on the way up, slow on the way down—making sure to keep your toes pointed upward. Lift your right thigh up until it's parallel to your left thigh; lower your right leg until your right heel is approximately one inch off the floor.

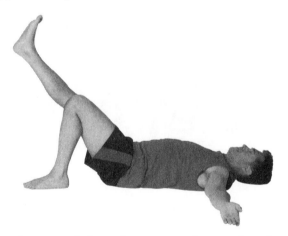

- Bring your leg up and down for a count of seven deep breaths in and out, then repeat with your opposite leg.

Adding the eccentric movement (braking contraction, or lowering of the leg) to this exercise significantly strengthens the lower abs. This exercise also targets the hip flexors, quadriceps, and hamstrings.

BOUND-ANGLE SEATED STRETCH

- Take a seated position on the floor with both knees bent. Slowly draw one foot at a time in toward your groin so that the soles of your feet are touching, forming a diamond with your lower body.
- Grab both feet and bring them toward your chest as you bend forward from your hips. Push down on your calves with your elbows as you bring your feet up.

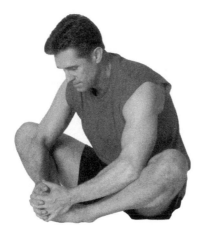

- You should feel a good stretch in your inner-thigh muscles and lower back. Hold for a count of seven deep breaths in and out.

This exercise provides a good stretch to your groin, hip, and lower-back muscles, increasing the range of motion in your hips so you can make a better turn behind the ball and through impact.

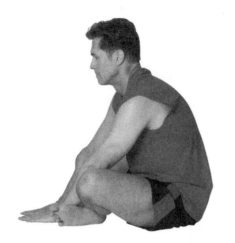 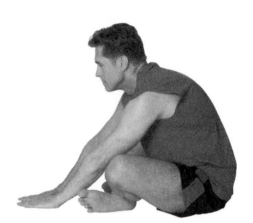

- Sit up on the floor in a simple cross-legged position, with both ankles touching the floor.
- Extend your arms out in front of you so that both palms are touching the floor.
- Reach forward with both hands as you bend forward from your hips, making sure to keep your neck in line with your spine. Hold for a count of seven deep breaths in and out.

This exercise improves your overall hip flexibility while also providing a good stretch for your lower back.

SIDE TREE SITTING UP

- Sit up on the floor with your left leg straight and your right knee bent. Cross your right leg over your left so that the outside of your right foot is touching the outside of your left knee.
- Take your left hand and wrap it around the outside of your right knee, then extend your right arm behind you so your right palm is flat on the floor.
- Holding your bent right knee in place, slowly twist your upper body to the right, looking back over your right shoulder as you turn your upper torso.

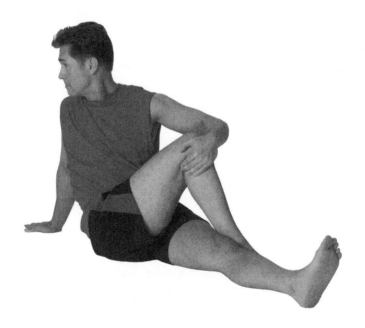

Twist as far as your range of motion will allow, then hold for a count of seven deep breaths in and out.
- Return to the starting position, then switch legs, this time twisting your upper body to your left. You should feel a good stretch in your buttocks, obliques, and lumbar spine.

BACK EXTENSION

- Lie on your stomach with your thighs and toes touching the floor and your elbows tucked under your shoulders, palms flat on the floor.

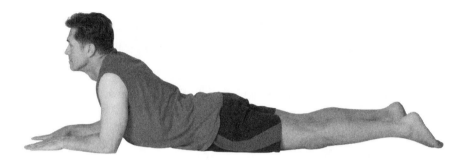

- Lengthen your legs out away from your hips, then slowly press your body backward so that your rib cage clears the floor. Feel like your shoulder blades are staying down and back as you bring your elbows off the floor.

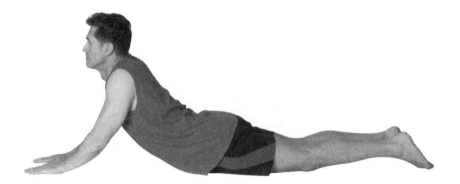

- Do not push up with your arms; allow them to straighten and support you as you lengthen your neck and hips.
- Hold the position for seven deep breaths in and out.

In addition to stretching your back, you'll gain some upper-body strength (in your shoulders) by bringing your elbows off the floor.

FLEXIBILITY PRAYER

- Stand up straight with your feet as wide as your shoulder blades and your arms hanging comfortably at your sides. Bring your arms up in front of you and join your hands together as though in prayer.
- Slowly twist your upper body to one side, allowing your hips to rotate some. Keep your arms and neck in one continuous straight line as you turn, trying to get your hands to finish directly behind you.
- Hold the position for seven deep breaths in and out, then slowly face front and repeat to the other side. You should feel a good stretch in your hip and back muscles as you engage your core.

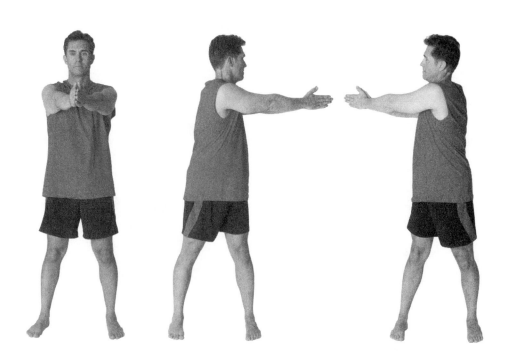

- Stand up straight with your arms extended diagonally out in front of you, at about a 45-degree angle, for balance.
- Kick your right leg directly out to the side and move it straight up and down—fast on the way up, slow on the way down. Inhale on the way up, and exhale very slowly on the way down.
- Make sure to line up the center of your forehead, chest, and navel with the inside of your left ankle as you push your leg out. This will prevent you from swaying too much with your lower body.
- Move your leg up and down for a count of seven deep breaths in and out. Return your right foot to the starting position, then repeat on the opposite leg for a good stretch on the outside of your hip.

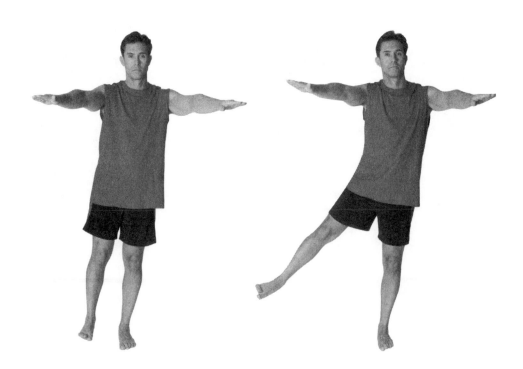

FINGERS TO TOES STANDING

- Stand up straight with your feet shoulder-width apart and your arms extended out to your sides, forming a letter "T."
- Slowly twist your upper body to the left as you touch the fingertips of your right hand to your left ankle.
- Look back at your left arm as you reach for your left foot, making sure to keep your belly button as low to the ground as possible.
- Hold the position for a count of seven deep breaths in and out and return to the starting position. Then reach your left hand toward your right foot.

This exercise will help improve your spinal rotation and increase your hamstring flexibility.

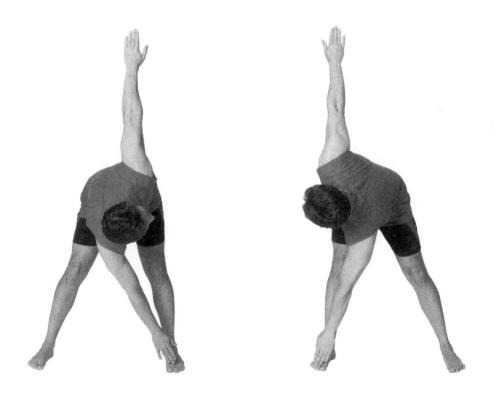

- Stand up straight with your arms down at your sides and your eyes fixed straight ahead. Bring your right foot up off the ground and place the sole of your foot up against the inside of your left knee.
- Slowly sweep your arms up above your head, gently pressing your right foot into your left knee as you reach for the sky.
- Hold for a count of seven deep breaths in and out. The center of your forehead, chest, and navel should all line up with the inside of your left ankle.
- Return to the starting position and repeat with your left foot joining the inside of your right knee.

This exercise will help improve your balance on the standing leg while also engaging your core muscles for support.

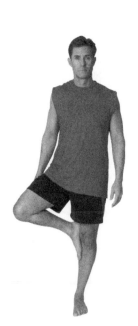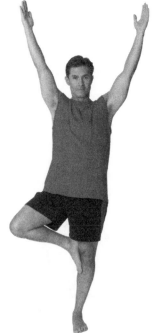

Congratulations! You've now completed *Golf Rx* Series B. To learn how to increase your stamina, proceed on to *Golf Rx* Series C.

CHAPTER FOURTEEN

INCREASING YOUR ENDURANCE:
GOLF Rx SERIES C

In baseball, Tiger Woods would be known as a premier closer. Forty times he has held or shared the fifty-four-hole lead in a PGA Tour event, and he's won thirty-seven times (through the 2006 PGA Championship). He's a perfect 12–0 with a fifty-four-hole lead in major championships.

Besides a fierce, competitive nature that rivals the likes of Michael Jordan and Wayne Gretzky, Woods's outstanding record can be attributed to his superb endurance. Tiger is as physically strong and mentally sharp on the 72nd hole of regulation as he is on the first. He never takes a hole off, grinding away to the very end even if he's far out of contention. Perhaps that explains why he made a record 142 consecutive cuts, a streak that spanned seven years.

This chapter focuses on building endurance, particularly in the core. It gives you the ability to fire a muscle over and over again at the same rate of speed, whether you're on the first tee or the 18th.

Hold each of these poses for ten full breaths.

- Lie flat on your back with your legs extended and your feet slightly turned out.
- Engage your abs by dropping your navel toward your spine, and raise your legs about twelve inches so your calves are no longer touching the floor.
- Reach your hands toward your knees and slowly bring your head off the floor, tucking your chin into your chest so you can look at your navel.
- Pump your arms up and down in a parallel fashion for a count of ten full breaths. Try to keep your arms in rhythm and the tips of your shoulder blades in contact with the floor. If you feel any neck tension, rest your head on a pillow.

Ultimately, you should be able to work up to a hundred total pumps (each up-and-down movement counts as one) for a complete core workout.

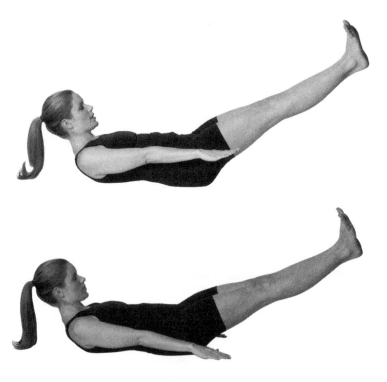

SUPINE LEG BEATS

- Lie flat on your back with your legs straight, feet slightly turned out, and hands behind your head to support your neck.

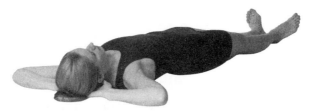

- Pull your navel in toward your spine to engage your abs, then slowly raise both legs several inches off the floor.

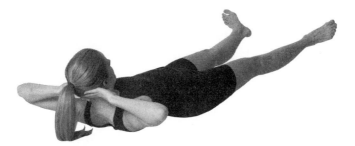

- Beat your heels together as you take ten full breaths in and out, allowing the weight of your legs to be supported by your lower abs. Keep lengthening the line between the base of your spine and your neck as you tap your heels together.

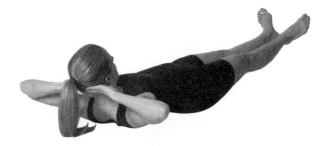

This exercise works the front and center of your core, in particular your lower abs.

- Lie flat on your back with your knees bent and your hands behind your head.
- Straighten your left leg, holding it at about a 45-degree angle, and bring your right knee toward your chest. As you do this, twist your left elbow toward the outside of your right knee. Alternately twist each elbow up toward the opposite knee, continuously moving your legs in a bicycle-like fashion.
- Try to keep your lower back flat on the floor and your elbows fanned out as much as possible. Continue to twist your torso and pedal your legs for a count of ten full breaths in and out.

This is a good strengthening exercise for your lower abs and oblique muscles. Keeping the thigh of your bent leg as straight as possible will force you to use your abs more.

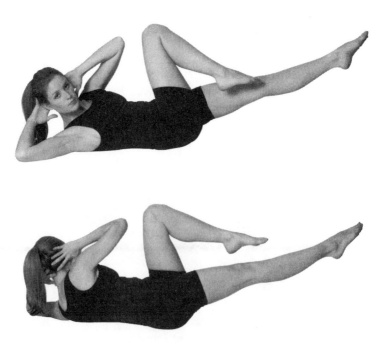

REVERSE CRUNCH

- Lie flat on your back with your arms straight at your sides and feet flat on the floor.
- Curl your knees up to your chest, then reach for the ceiling with the balls of your feet. Lift your tailbone off the floor by using your lower abs.
- Remember to keep your knees over your chest and make sure to press your lower back into the floor throughout the exercise. Continue to drive your feet toward the ceiling, taking ten full breaths in and out.

This exercise strengthens your lower abs, which provide support to the lower back, and your trunk muscles (hip flexors and extensors).

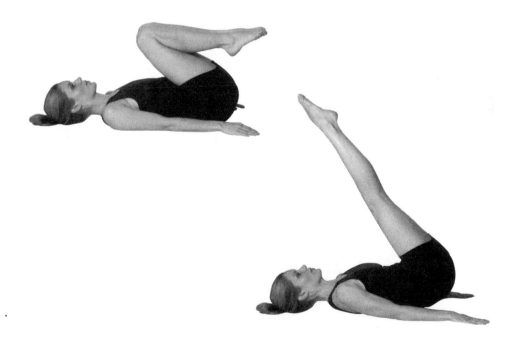

CIRCLES

- Lie flat on your back with both legs straight, toes pointing straight ahead.
- Bring your right leg up into a straight position, then circle the leg around in a counterclockwise circular motion as though you were tracing your toes around a clock, with midnight being directly above your nose.

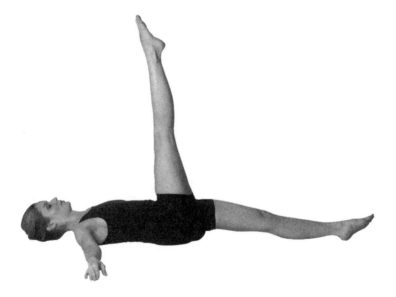

- Swing your leg up, around, and across your body, quickly on the way up and slowly on the way down. Continue circling the leg around for ten full breaths, inhaling and exhaling with each circle. Then repeat with the opposite leg, keeping your lower back on the floor and your hips even with the floor.

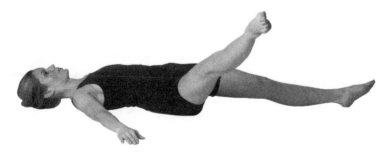

- Resisting the movement on the way down helps to strengthen your hamstrings and buttocks, while the quicker upward movements help to lengthen your hamstrings.

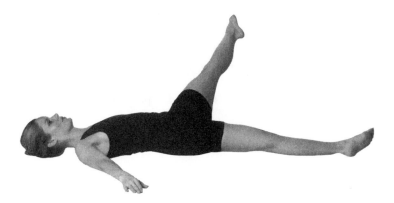

- Lie flat on your back with your legs bent and arms extended out to the sides, forming a "T."
- Cross your right leg over your bent left knee so that it's in contact with the outside of your knee.
- Use the weight of your right leg to apply pressure to the outside of your left knee, bringing it to the floor. Increase the pressure to your left leg by pulling your right leg down with your right hand.
- Hold the stretch for at least ten deep breaths and then return to the starting position, with both knees bent.
- Repeat with the opposite leg to help increase the internal rotation of your hips, which is pivotal for reducing the stress on your lower back in the follow-through.

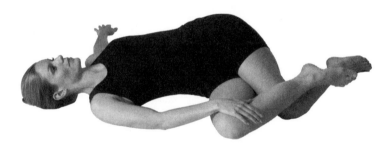

UPWARD-FACING DOG

- Lie on your stomach with your toes pointed straight back and your arms tucked under your shoulders, with your palms and forearms flat on the floor.

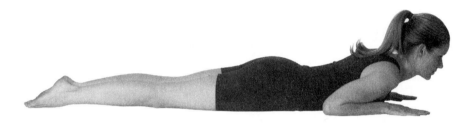

- Feel as though you are lengthening your legs away from your hips, then slowly raise your upper body just enough so that the base of your ribs come off the floor.

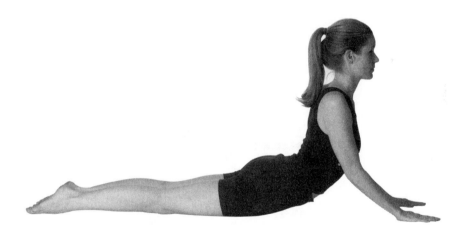

- Allow your arms to support you, but don't push up with them. Keep your neck relaxed and your shoulder blades down and back.
- Hold the position for a count of ten deep breaths in and out to help build endurance in the extensor muscles of your lower back.

- Lie flat on your stomach with your heels touching, toes pointed straight back, and your hands folded underneath your forehead.
- Keeping your hands on your forehead, raise both legs together about six inches off of the ground. You can place a pillow under your belly for additional support.
- Tap the insides of your heels together, keeping the movement fairly rapid as you take ten deep breaths in and out. Keep lengthening the line between the base of your spine and your neck as you tap your heels together.

This exercise builds endurance in your lower-back muscles and also works your hip abductors and adductors.

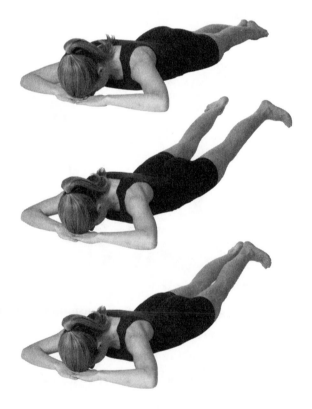

STANDING FINGERS TO TOES

- Stand up straight with your feet shoulder-width apart and arms extended out to your sides, forming a letter "T."
- Slowly twist your upper body to the right as you reach your left hand toward your right foot. Try and get your fingertips to touch your toes or the floor.
- Look back at your right arm as you reach for your right foot, making sure to keep your belly button as low to the ground as possible. Do not lift your head or chest to see your hand.
- Hold the position for a count of ten deep breaths in and out and return to the starting position. Then reach your right hand toward your left foot.

This exercise increases your spinal rotation and hamstring flexibility.

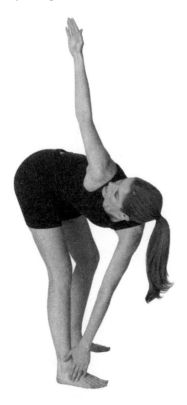

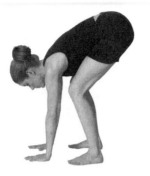

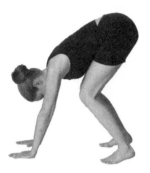

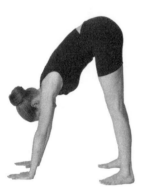

- From a standing position, bend your knees and bring your hands down to the floor.
- Walk your hands out away from you until you feel most of your body weight being absorbed by your hands. Distribute your weight evenly on both hands.
- Allow your head to hang as though it's a cherry on a stem, and relax your back. Next, alternately straighten and bend your knees for a count of ten deep breaths in and out. As you straighten your knees, your buttocks should move closer to the ceiling.

This exercise strengthens the quads (you should feel a strong burn there toward the end of the exercise) and lengthens the top part of your hamstrings. It also stretches and loosens up your lower back.

DOWNWARD-FACING DOG

- Assume a push-up position (hands and feet shoulder-width apart) with your weight evenly distributed on your hands and toes.
- Walk your feet in as close to your hands as possible, so that your body forms an inverted "V." Relax your weight into your hands and feet and let your head hang as you walk your feet forward.
- You should feel a good stretch in your calves and hamstrings. Try to keep your feet flat on the floor, but if you can't, start out in a wider "V" and gradually work your way forward until you can hold your heels down.
- Hold for a count of ten full breaths in and out.

This exercise is great for lengthening your calves and hamstrings, and it targets your entire core. It also builds strength in your arms and shoulders.

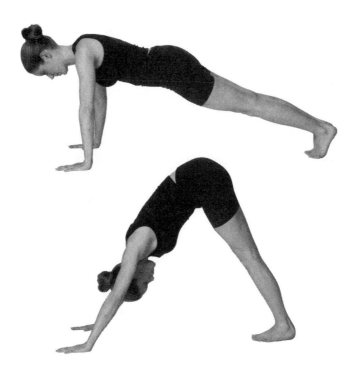

- Stand on one leg with the opposite leg slightly bent.
- Reach across your body diagonally to try to throw off your balance. As you get more comfortable with the exercise, you can reach across farther and/or quicker.
- Hold for a count of ten deep breaths in and out, return to the starting position, and then switch legs.
- Feel as though the hip on your standing leg is lifted and tall.

This exercise increases your awareness, or feel, for your hips, knees, and ankles relative to the other parts of your body. This builds sturdiness in the standing leg at the bookends (top of backswing and finish) of your swing.

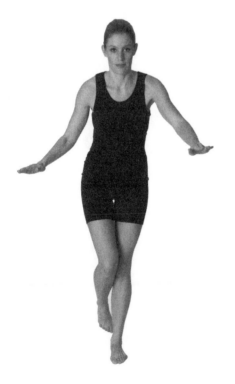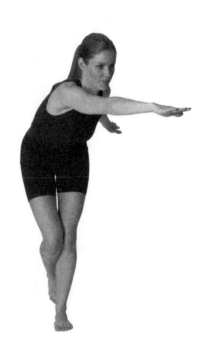

STANDING TWIST WITH SHOULDER STRETCH

- Stand up straight with your feet the same width apart as your shoulder blades.
- Extend your left arm out in front of you and place the back of your right hand, palm facing forward, against your forearm (just in front of your elbow).
- Using your right hand, gently pull your left arm across your chest toward your right shoulder until you feel a stretch at the back of your left shoulder. At the same time, slowly twist your torso to the right until your left thumb is behind you.
- Keep your toes and knees facing forward as you turn and keep your arms and neck in one continuous straight line. Hold for a count of ten full breaths in and out, then repeat on the other side to stretch the posterior muscles in your shoulders and the paraspinal muscles in your back. Both muscle groups help in the deceleration, or braking, phase of the swing to protect your shoulders and lower back from injury.

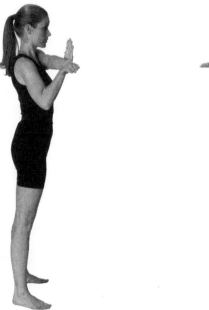 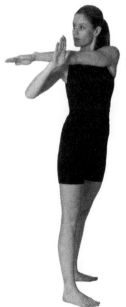

- Stand up straight with your arms extended diagonally out in front you, at about a 45-degree angle, for balance.
- Lift your right leg directly out to the side until you feel a good stretch on the outside of your right hip. Instead of holding the foot in place, however, loop it around in a circle for a count of ten deep breaths in and out.
- Return to the starting position and repeat with the opposite leg.
- Make sure to line up the center of your forehead, chest, and navel with the inside ankle of your standing leg. Feel as though the hip on your standing leg is lifted and tall, as if it were up against a wall. This will prevent the hip from sliding out.

This exercise strengthens the hip-abductor muscles, which are very important in kick-starting the swing and building torque in your backswing.

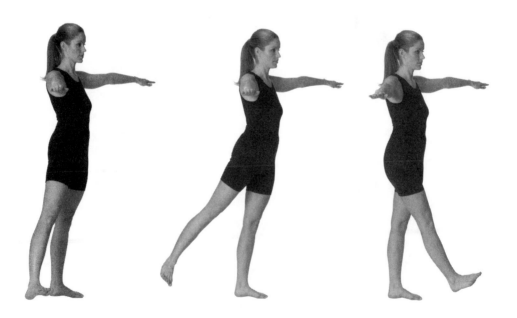

ADVANCED TREE POSE

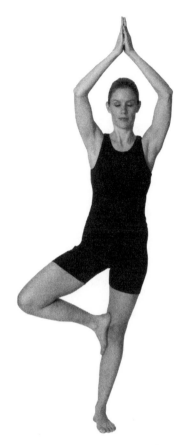

- Stand up straight with your arms down at your sides and your neck acting as one long extension of your spine. Bring your right foot up and place the sole of the foot against the inside of your left knee.
- Slowly sweep your arms up above your head and join your hands as though in prayer, gently pressing your right foot into your left knee as you reach for the sky.
- Close your eyes and hold for a count of ten deep breaths in and out, looking to your core to help provide balance.
- Return to the starting position and repeat with your left foot joining the inside of your right knee. Try to keep the center of your forehead, chest, and navel in a straight line with the inside of your standing ankle.

This exercise will help improve your balance on your standing leg while also engaging your core muscles for support.

Congratulations! You've now completed *Golf Rx* Series C. For additional strength and endurance exercises, see Chapter Four. To learn more about the most common golf-related injuries and how to treat them, proceed on to Part Three and Chapter Fifteen.

PART THREE

INJURY PREVENTION
AND CARE

LOWER-BACK PAIN:
GOLF'S GREATEST HANDICAP

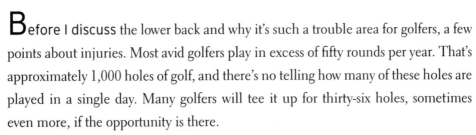

Before I discuss the lower back and why it's such a trouble area for golfers, a few points about injuries. Most avid golfers play in excess of fifty rounds per year. That's approximately 1,000 holes of golf, and there's no telling how many of these holes are played in a single day. Many golfers will tee it up for thirty-six holes, sometimes even more, if the opportunity is there.

This addiction to the game can be dangerous if your body is not conditioned to play so much golf. The majority of golf injuries—approximately 80 percent—are overuse injuries. These injuries are mostly seen in the back, but they can also occur in the shoulder, elbow, hip, and knee. The underlying cause of these injuries is a loss of flexibility, strength, and endurance in your core muscle group, which the exercises in *Golf Rx* are designed to counteract.

Improper swing technique is the second-biggest cause of golf injuries. An abbreviated finish or sudden stop (rapid deceleration) of the club can cause harm to the wrists, elbows, shoulders, hips, and back. To improve your swing mechanics and build a swing that is less likely to cause you pain, please refer back to Chapter One.

Rapid golf progression after being "golf-deconditioned" during the off-season can also cause injuries. This rapid progression to golf—from sitting on the couch regularly to teeing it up on the first day of the new season—is the third-most common cause of injury. In the ten years I've been practicing, I've treated more than 3,000 golfers at every level—professional, amateur, and recreational. I'd estimate that half of these golfers came to me early in the season, usually with a lower-back injury.

Your body has been golf-deconditioned since you last played several months ago, and it needs to be brought back slowly. *Golf Rx* will keep your core conditioned and fit to play, so that when the season rolls around, you'll be able to go immediately without fear of injury.

Inherent anatomical factors, such as a low clearance between the humeral head and acromion in the shoulder and the ulna and carpal bones in the wrist, can also put you at risk for injury (more on this in Chapter Sixteen). Lastly, there are extraneous factors such as flying, smoking, dehydration, and obesity. The latter is a major contributor to lower-back, knee, and ankle injuries, because the more weight you carry, the more pressure you put on these extremities during the swing.

In this chapter, I'm going to focus solely on lower-back injuries, the most common form of injury suffered by recreational and professional golfers. It is estimated that half of all recreational golfers and one-third of all professional golfers suffer from some form of lower-back pain. The primary cause, as we learned from our study of forty-two PGA Tour golfers at the 2001 Buick Classic, is a lack of flexibility (range of motion) in the lead hip, or the left hip for right-handed golfers. As soon as the ball is hit, the body goes into a rapid slowdown mode, and if the primary shock absorbers (hips, lower-back muscles, and glutes) are fatigued and not working properly, the lower back takes on too much stress. The joints, disks, and supporting structures wear down, often cutting your season short before it even begins.

FACET JOINT PAIN

Consider: The average golf swing takes under two seconds to complete. More than half of that time elapses between the start of the swing and impact. This means that from the moment of impact, you have just a few tenths of a second to bring a club traveling from 70 to 100-plus miles per hour to a complete stop. That's less time than it takes most people to remove a headcover.

A strong, well-conditioned core will help dissipate this speed so your back doesn't take on too much stress in the rapid deceleration, or braking, phase of the swing. But if the core is fatigued, weak, or not functioning properly, the back takes on too much load. In the professional golfers we tested, a loss of internal rotation in the lead hip was the primary cause of their lower-back problems. Loss of this internal rotation of the hip causes the joints and disks in the lower back to absorb too much stress as the club slows down.

The segment of the back most prone to injury or acute pain with golfers is the facet joint. Located two finger-widths away on each side of your spinal column, these joints are responsible for the flexion (bending forward), extension (bending backward), and rotation of the spine. They also serve as a braking mechanism, preventing the spine from turning too far.

Each facet joint is contained in a synovial capsule, which allows the joints to glide nicely against each other. Repeated swings, or overuse, along with muscle fatigue can put too much stress on these joints, causing the shock-absorbing synovial lining to become inflamed. This inflammation can cause some golfers to experience acute pain that radiates down into their buttocks.

With a facet injury, pain generally gets worse with walking and standing. You're not able to straighten up or stand for a long period of time.

Arthritis of the L4-5 facet joint of the spine is the most common arthritic condition in recreational and professional golfers. For right-handed players, it is the right L4-5 that is most commonly involved. The L4-5 level is exposed to a lot of torque loads during the swing. This leads to repeated use of the L4-5 facet joint.

I have seen many professional golfers—some in their late twenties—who have early arthritis of the L4-5 joint due to overuse. And the problem only gets worse as you get older and lose the cushion between the L4 and L5 vertebrae, known as the disk. The wearing down of this disk puts even more torque loads on the facet joint. This type of arthritis is most commonly seen in fifty-five- to sixty-five-year-old golfers, because they have lost some disk space that predisposes their L4-5 joint to additional wear and tear. *Golf Rx* minimizes torque loads on the L4-5 joint by restoring flexibility, strength, and endurance.

Typically, golfers with arthritis of the L4-5 facet joint will complain of back and buttock pain that is worsened with prolonged standing or walking. The condition is treated by doing stretches like Series A in *Back Rx* combined with bicycling, use of anti-inflammatories, and icing the back every morning. If that doesn't work, facet-joint injections or a procedure called radiofrequency denervation must be done.

BATTLE OF THE BULGE

The other common lower-back injury in golf is the bulging disk. This occurs when shear stresses—often, the result of too much wear and tear—are placed on the front of the disk, causing the soft material in the disk's nucleus to bulge backward like jelly oozing out of a donut. This internal material, also known as nucleus pulposus, often spills into a nerve, causing acute pain in the lower back that gets worse with sitting and bending forward.

A disk that's worn out or bulging is like a car that encounters a series of bumps with no shock absorbers. There's nothing to absorb the forces between the adjacent vertebrae, so the joints feel more jarring with physical activity.

ICING AND OTHER PREVENTIVE MEASURES

At the first onset of lower-back pain, ice your back just before going to bed. While lying on the floor, prop your feet up on a chair so your legs are bent at a 90-degree angle and place an ice pack under your lower back. Lie in this position for fifteen minutes. Also, take two to three Advil during lunch and dinner for the first day or two, if it's not contraindicated and has been cleared by your physician. If the pain persists for more than five days, see a doctor. (For more on how to treat a facet-joint injury to your lower back, see the case study in Chapter Eighteen.)

Starting an exercise program like *Golf Rx* will help reduce the likelihood of your incurring a lower-back injury. The exercises in Series A, B, and C are designed to bring more flexibility, strength, and endurance to your core so you can lessen the impact of the swing on your back. The following are some other preventive methods you can take in the fight against lower-back pain.

- If you have a desk job, make sure to get up once every thirty minutes to an hour. Stroll to the water cooler or, if you prefer to stand, rest your hands on your hips, positioning your thumbs in line with the paraspinal muscles that extend up and down both sides of your spine. Slowly arch your back backward. Hold this position for thirty seconds to lengthen your hips and take some pressure off your disks.
- When sitting at your desk, consider propping your feet up on a phone book. This puts your back into slight extension, which relieves pressure on the disks. Do not lean forward at your desk, because this also puts too much stress on the disks.
- When sleeping, rest on your side in a fetal position—not on your stomach or back. When you sleep on your back, your weight tends to push down on

the mattress, which flexes your back and puts extra pressure on the disks. On your stomach, your back goes into extension, which, over the course of seven or eight hours, is bad for your joints. Lying on your side takes pressure off the disks and joints.

- If you frequently fly for business, take two or three anti-inflammatory tablets such as Advil (if it's not contraindicated and has been cleared by your physician) with lunch and dinner to help minimize inflammation on the joints and disks. The pressurized cabin and low oxygen levels on the plane, combined with prolonged sitting, puts you at great risk for a herniated disk or other lower-back injury, especially if you plan to play golf shortly after exiting the plane.

LOWER-BACK PAIN FIRST-AID CHEST

What do you do if you're in pain right now? Follow these simple steps to ease your pain and begin your healing.

1. Focus on and regulate your breathing. Proper breathing in a slow, controlled rhythm is the fastest pain reliever you can use. It shifts the mind's attention away from the pain and triggers the body's natural relaxation response.

     Lie flat on the floor on your back with your knees up and your lower legs resting on a chair, or some pillows, or lie on your side in a fetal position with a pillow between your knees. Let your body guide you into the least painful position possible.

     Slow down your breathing as much as possible. Exhale fully, then inhale deeply and hold the breath in your lungs for a count of three. Exhale fully, and continue breathing this way for at least two to three minutes.

     Repeat this process throughout the day to calm yourself and to deliver extra oxygen to overstressed muscles and disks, allowing them to begin to relax, breathe, and take in nourishment.

2. Take anti-inflammatory and pain-relief medication to speed healing. The most readily available over-the-counter pain-relief medicines are aspirin, ibuprofen (Advil), and acetaminophen (Tylenol). Ibuprofen is generally the best choice for lower-back pain, because unlike acetaminophen, it provides anti-inflammatory as well as pain-relief benefits.

3. Take modified bed rest for two to three days. Spend most of the day resting quietly in the most comfortable position you can find. The two positions that work best for most people are on the side in a slightly fetal position with a pillow between the knees, or flat on the back with the legs raised. The second position really encourages the lower-back muscles to relax because it takes all the strain of gravity off them.

4. Hit the water. If you have access to a pool, aquatherapy can speed your recovery. Your buoyancy in the water will take all the pressure off the lower back.

5. Apply ice. In the first twenty-four to forty-eight hours after a lower-back injury, apply ice to tender areas two to three times a day for ten to fifteen minutes at a time in order to lessen inflammation. Keeping the ice on for longer won't give you any added benefit; it reaches its maximum efficacy after about ten minutes.

6. Add heat. After twenty-four hours apply moist heat in the shower or with a heating pad for up to thirty minutes at a time, as desired. Unlike cold, gentle warmth may continue to provide an increased benefit if it is applied for a longer period of time.

CHAPTER SIXTEEN

OTHER COMMON GOLF INJURIES: UPPER EXTREMITIES

Sometimes, the golf course is the safest place for a professional golfer. Case in point: Tom Lehman. The 1996 British Open winner nearly missed the 1998 Open championship when he hurt his right shoulder playing with his kids at an amusement park, just two days prior to the start of the event. Only much later did he learn that he had separated his shoulder, which would require surgery in the off-season. "They said it [my shoulder] looked like the shoulder of a guy who had been playing in the NFL for ten years," said Lehman, whose shoulder joint had deteriorated to the point that it looked like a mangled golf ball.

Retief Goosen had to withdraw from the 2004 PGA Championship after he injured his hip falling off a Jet Ski in Barbados. Fellow South African Ernie Els didn't fare so well on the open water either, rupturing the anterior cruciate ligament in his left knee while on a sailing vacation in the Mediterranean in July 2005. Els wound up missing the remainder of the PGA Tour season.

Excluding falls and bizarre injuries such as these, the following are several common golf injuries you'll find in the upper extremities of the body.

NECK INJURIES: STRAINS AND OTHER PAINS

If you watch LPGA Hall of Famer Annika Sorenstam swing, it looks as though her head is on a swivel. Her head rotates in sync with her upper body so quickly that it appears as though she's looking straight ahead at the target at impact, not at the ball. While most golfers don't rotate their heads as fluidly as Annika, they do turn their heads to see the ball and the target. In some instances, the head changes direction very abruptly from the top of the backswing to the forward swing. Other golfers try to keep their head completely still while rotating the rest of their body. These types of movements put additional strain and load on the neck, making it more susceptible to injury.

The cervical spine, which begins at the base of the neck, is far less prone to injury than the lower lumbar spine or thoracic spine (mid- and upper back). In most instances, the neck is the victim, not the culprit.

"If a golfer is complaining about neck pain, he should start from the ground and work his way up to find the culprit," says Stanley A. Herring, M.D., Medical Director of Spine Care at the University of Washington in Seattle, and also a team physician for the Seattle Seahawks football team. "Generally, the problem is elsewhere.

"In an ideal swing, you want your body to face the target or slightly left of the target at the finish," says Herring. "If you have a bad back or a sore hip, you'll open your shoulders and cervical spine early so you can see the ball sooner. The neck changes its normal course of motion, and that's how it gets hurt."

Trying to keep your head still while other muscles are contracting around it also puts more shear forces on the neck and can put your cervical spine at risk. Most neck injuries in golf involve strains to the ligaments, tendons, and muscles that help support and stabilize the cervical spine. Due to disk shrinkage (i.e., a loss of water content), older golfers are more likely to rupture, or herniate, a disk in their neck. The problem is exacerbated by trying to keep your head still, which forces the disks to remain stationary while your body is shifting and rotating. This puts tremendous strain on the disks.

Business travelers are predisposed to this injury because of the pressurized cabin and low oxygen levels on an airplane. If a disk hasn't been oxygenated properly, it's at a high risk of bulging. Again, to use the jelly-donut analogy, too much pressure is applied to the front of the disk, causing the inner jelly to ooze backward into the spinal column where nerves are present.

Make sure to stretch your neck gently before you play (see Chapter Six to learn how). It's very easy to overlook the neck because it's not part of your core, but it needs to be stretched regularly, just like your hamstrings, hips, and lower back. The neck also loves heat, so if you've experienced some stiffness in your neck before or if you fly frequently, apply a heating pad to it for fifteen minutes before you go to bed.

SHOULDER INJURIES: ROTATOR-CUFF PROBLEMS

Most shoulder injuries in golf involve the rotator cuff—a group of four muscles and connective tendons that attach to the top of the humerus bone (the long arm bone that connects the shoulder to the elbow). These muscles are extremely important to the proper functioning of the golf swing, because they allow you to lift your arms up over your head and rotate them toward and away from your body. They also work together to support the ligaments and stabilize the shoulder joint.

Some golfers are predisposed to rotator-cuff tendinitis, especially early on, because of an increased laxity, or elasticity, in the capsule that surrounds the front of the shoulder joint. The capsule stabilizes the joint, keeping the ball in the socket. With repetitive use, the front capsule becomes even looser and more unstable, which can cause the humeral head to slip out the front of the shoulder; it can also slide down the back or to the bottom—a condition known as multidirectional instability.

"If the shoulder joint is inherently unstable, it's been described as trying to balance a beach ball on a seal's nose," says James R. Andrews, M.D., a founding member of the Alabama Sports Medicine and Orthopedic Center in Birmingham, Alabama, and the official medical director for the LPGA Tour. "It's hard to keep the shoulder joint in the socket."

The rotator cuff must work overtime to hold the shoulder joint in place, says Andrews, and it therefore gets overused, causing the tendinitis. This is most commonly seen in the lead, or left, shoulder, of right-handed golfers. The shoulder becomes so painful that you can't play.

The best way to prevent such an injury is to strengthen the rotator-cuff muscles (see Chapter Four for a rotator cuff–specific stretch) and scapular stabilizers, which will help to keep the humerus from sliding out the front of the shoulder. You also want to stretch the posterior capsule and the muscles at the back of your shoulder to prevent them from getting too tight. This simple shoulder stretch will accomplish it: Lie on your back and reach your right arm across your chest, then gently pull your right elbow farther across your chest with your left hand, toward your left shoulder. Hold for a count of ten deep breaths in and out and repeat with your opposite arm. You can also perform this stretch standing, using the back of your wrist to pull the opposite arm across your body.

Older golfers are more likely to develop rotator-cuff tendinitis with impingement. This occurs when the humerus bone in your upper arm rides up into the acromion bone, which lies on top of the rotator cuff, pinching the cuff in between. The two bones come together and the rotator cuff gets caught in the middle, causing it to fray or tear and making it extremely painful to lift your arms overhead. You'll not only have a difficult time turning your arms and shoulders to the top of the swing, but you'll have trouble braking your swing and completing your follow-through.

ELBOW INJURIES: TENNIS AND GOLFER'S ELBOW

The repeated bending of the wrists caused by the hinging and unhinging of the club puts a great deal of stress on the elbows. At no time is this greater than in the impact zone, when the wrists are unhinging and the clubshaft is catching up to the left (lead) arm and reaching its maximum speed. The wrists whip the clubhead through the ball, and this generates a tremendous amount of force when your arms, body, and club are all synchronized correctly.

Repetitive stresses on the wrists and the muscles of the forearm can lead to one of two degenerative conditions—golfer's elbow or tennis elbow. People who suffer from golfer's elbow, also known as medial epicondylitis, will experience discomfort on the inside part of the elbow, whereas those with tennis elbow (lateral epicondylitis) will experience pain on the outside of the elbow joint.

If your arms are relaxed at your sides, palms turned inward, the outside of your elbow is farthest from your body, whereas the inside part is touching your body.

With golfer's elbow, the pain worsens when you flex your wrist or pull your palm toward you. With tennis elbow, the pain worsens with overuse of the extensor muscles on the outside of your forearm—those muscles that pull your wrist away from you (i.e., bend the wrist backward). Ironically, you'll see more cases of tennis elbow in golfers than golfer's elbow, says Robert Marx, M.D., an orthopedic surgeon based at the Hospital for Special Surgery in New York.

"Tennis elbow is more common because of the way we use our arms," says Marx. "We tend to extend them outward, away from our body. It's the opposite of curling a straight barbell: We don't pull our arms in. Everything is out in front of us."

Poorly fitted clubs (i.e., swinging a club that's too heavy or too stiff) can also lead to tennis elbow, says Marx. If the club is too heavy, it's going to put a lot of pressure on the outside of the elbow, especially as the clubhead approaches impact. Typically, if a club is too heavy or stiff, you'll have a hard time turning the clubface over, and you'll hit a lot of shots low and to the right. But to really know for sure, go see your local clubfitter.

You want to make sure your grip fits your palm, too, says James Andrews, who also serves as the senior orthopedic consultant for the Washington Redskins football team. A grip that's too thin will cause you to hold the club too tightly; conversely, one that's too big will force you to hold it lightly. When you grip the club, the two middle fingers of your left hand should gently touch the thumb pad of your left hand. They should not dig into your thumb pad or fall short of it.

Much like the neck, the elbows are frequently overlooked when it comes to stretching. Make sure to stretch your wrist flexors and extensors (see "Elbow and Wrist Stretch" in Chapter Six) regularly to maintain good flexibility in your elbow joints.

WRIST INJURIES: TFC TEARS AND TENDINITIS

At the point of impact (with an iron), all of your weight is being loaded onto the shaft, and the clubhead is descending down into the ball and the turf. The clubhead contacts the ball and then cuts a divot on the target side of the ball. In some instances, when hitting out of high grass or fluffy sand, or even off a hard, bare surface, the clubhead will come to a sudden stop with little or no follow-through. There's no give to the hitting surface, which can cause tears and other types of damage to your left wrist (the lead wrist for right-handed golfers).

The most common of these "impact" injuries is a tear to the triangular fibrocartilage complex (TFC), which sits in a small space between the carpal (wrist) bones and the ulna bone at the end of your forearm—on the side opposite your thumb. Jim Furyk underwent surgery to repair this cartilage in March 2004, nine months after he won his first U.S. Open championship. Furyk had experienced pain in his left wrist for years, pain he said grew worse when he practiced on firm ground like the players see at the British Open.

The repetitive strain on the left wrist through impact is what led to Furyk's injury. The wrist is not a weight-bearing joint, so it's not conditioned to handle the trauma that impact—and the whiplash-like motion the lead wrist experiences through the ball—can sometimes cause.

Another cause of TFC tears is a low-riding ulna. Some people are born with this condition, in which the ulna rides too far down into the wrist joint, toward your knuckles. If the separation between the ulna and carpal bones is too low, it can lead to a tear of the TFC.

If you regularly feel discomfort at impact or when you use your lead wrist to shake hands, you should stop playing immediately and go see a doctor. Another way to diagnose a TFC problem is to perform Finkelstein's test: Make a fist so the fingers of your left hand curl over your thumb, and then push your wrist downward toward your pinky. If there's tendinitis in the TFC or a tear, you will feel a lot of pain just under the bony projection at the end of the ulna.

The second-most common wrist injury in golf can also be detected using Finkelstein's test. It's known as De Quervain's tenosynovitis, and it results from the repetitive loading, or hinging, of the club upward during the swing. Golfers with this type of injury will feel some tenderness just above the thumb on the side of their hand (the one being hinged) where the forearm and wrist converge.

As with the elbow, make sure to stretch your wrist flexors and extensors regularly to avoid these problems. If you're hitting from tall grass, consider pitching the ball back to the fairway with your sand wedge or another high-lofted club. Don't try and force the ball out with a mid-iron, because the grass is likely to grab and twist the clubface and possibly injure your wrists.

CHAPTER SEVENTEEN

OTHER COMMON GOLF INJURIES: LOWER EXTREMITIES

In 2004, everyone in the golf world was asking, "What's wrong with Tiger Woods?" The man who was nearly invincible from 1999 through 2002, winning seven majors, including four in a row in one stretch (dubbed "The Tiger Slam"), suddenly couldn't win a golf tournament. He had split with his longtime swing coach, Butch Harmon, at the start of the 2003 season and had begun a second major swing renovation under the tutelage of Hank Haney. This also had people scratching their heads. Why, after such a dominating run, would Tiger change his swing . . . again? (Tiger first retooled his swing with Harmon after winning the 1997 Masters by twelve strokes.)

One reason why Tiger opted to change was because his old swing was damaging his left knee, to the extent that Woods had surgery on the knee after the 2002 season. Doctors removed fluid and a cyst from the knee, and also found that his anterior cruciate ligament, which is responsible for keeping the top bone of the knee from sliding forward and helps to stabilize the knee during sports activities such as soccer, was significantly stretched. Tiger, in his words, used to "snap his left leg straight" to gain a little extra power with his longer clubs. But that move, along with the power he generated from having such fast hips on the downswing, put too much stress on the knee. The pain got so bad in 2002 that Woods told *Golf Digest* magazine that in addition to taking pre-round painkillers, he would "move away from the ball" on the downswing to avoid putting pressure on his left knee.

KNEE INJURIES: MENISCUS TEARS

As Woods's history shows, the left leg—or lead leg for right-handed golfers—is a prime target for injury. The left knee joint is constantly twisting during the swing, in addition to bearing a lot of the body's weight and momentum. At the start of the downswing, the majority of your weight shifts to your left leg. The leg plants, creating a firm post—or axis point—for your hips and body to rotate around. Your right side fires through and, at the completion of the swing, nearly all of your weight is on your left leg.

Because the leg is repeatedly planting and twisting, the lead knee is very prone to meniscal tears and arthritis. The meniscus is a fibrous pad that sits between the femur (thigh bone) and tibia (large bone in lower leg) within the knee and helps minimize stresses on the articular cartilage, a tough, elastic tissue that covers the surface of the joint and allows the bones to glide smoothly over each another. "Excessive torque across the flexed knee can trap the meniscus between the two surfaces of the joint and cause a tear," says Answorth Allen, M.D., team physician for the New York Knicks basketball team. "Pain ranges from an ache to a sharp, catching pain that occurs with twisting motions."

Loss of this articular cartilage is what leads to arthritis in the knee joint. A lack of balance, the result of poor swing mechanics and frequent walking on uneven surfaces, also makes a golfer susceptible to meniscal tears. Your body is unable to make the micro-adjustments it needs to in time to restore balance to the knee, which puts additional stresses on the knee. This is why it's good to do exercises standing on one leg (see the "Standing Tree Pose" exercises in Series A, B, and C). These exercises help build proprioception in the knee, meaning your body will be able to recognize its individual components in space and make the necessary adjustments to keep your knee stable. This, in turn, will help prevent your meniscus from tearing.

HIPS: LABRAL TEARS

The hip is the largest joint in the human body, and perhaps the most important in the golf swing. The ball and socket joint is responsible for rotating your lower body, as well as for moving it forward, backward, and from side to side. Its most important function is to rotate your lead hip internally after impact, so that it can help absorb some of the forces being thrown at your lower back as the swing comes to a stop.

Because it serves so many functions, it's very susceptible to overuse injuries. Younger golfers are prone to labral tears, older players to arthritis. The labrum is a shock-absorbing fibrous cartilage, much like the meniscus in the knee joint, that surrounds the outer rim of the hip socket and protects the articular cartilage that lines the bones of the joint. "Excessive torque across the joint can cause the labrum to be trapped between the femoral head and the socket, resulting in a tear," says Struan H. Coleman, M.D., Ph.D., an orthopedic surgeon with the Department of Sports Medicine and Shoulder Service at the Hospital for Special Surgery, and team physician for the New York Mets baseball team. "Symptoms range from an ache to a sharp, catching pain, and is usually localized to the groin. The patient will experience this pain with twisting motions such as the golf swing, or with more common activities such as climbing in and out of a car."

Older players are more likely to suffer from arthritis in the hip joint. Your joint is surrounded by a watertight sac, or capsule. Repeated hip motion in the golf swing causes the capsule to shrink, leaving little room for the joint to rotate. The hip loses some range of motion, putting more stress on the joint and cartilage and wearing the cartilage down.

Because of our sedentary lifestyles, all golfers are at a high risk for hip arthritis if they don't start a program like *Golf Rx* and stretch out their hip flexors and internal and external hip rotators. It is imperative to warm up and stretch before a round (see pre-round stretches in Chapter Five, several of which target your hips). "Failure to do so may result in injuries that will affect not just a golfer's handicap, but the ability to lead a normal life," says Dr. Coleman.

FOOT AND ANKLE: THE NEED FOR ORTHOTICS

On average, our feet log about 1,000 miles per year, or roughly the distance from New York City to Orlando, says Rock Positano, DPM, a foot and ankle specialist at the Hospital for Special Surgery in New York. A relatively active person takes about 6,000 steps per day, or roughly 2,000 steps every mile. When you consider that one mile equals 1,760 yards, and most eighteen-hole courses being walked today are 6,000-plus yards, that's roughly 7,000 steps per round of golf. And that's not factoring in the additional distance you have to walk to search for your golf ball, or the amount of time you spend standing on your feet. In other words, your feet take about as much of a pounding during the course of eighteen holes as your Titleist Pro V1 golf ball does.

Unfortunately, golf shoes are not built like running shoes. They're designed to give your feet better traction, not to cushion or support your feet. As a result, it's very common to see golfers with heel pain and inflammation of the plantar fascia, otherwise known as plantar fasciitis. The plantar fascia is a thick connective tissue on the underside of your foot. People with plantar fasciitis generally experience pain in the front and back of the heel akin to stepping on a pebble barefoot. The pain tends to be most severe with the first step in the morning. Overweight people have the greatest chance of incurring plantar fasciitis, although repetitive walking and standing in poorly cushioned golf shoes can also put you at high risk.

The second-most common foot or ankle injury in golf is Achilles tendinitis. Inflammation of the Achilles tendon, which is the largest in the human body, is common among athletes who spend a lot of time on their feet. The golf course, with its rolling hills and sidehill lies, invites even more trouble. Walking and hitting balls off of so many uneven lies puts additional strain on the tendon. Generally, the worst pain is felt an inch to two above the point where the tendon attaches to your heel bone.

Lastly, you can develop arthritis in your ankle or big toe. If you feel some tenderness in your heel, it's a good idea to stretch your fascia before you go to bed. You can stretch it by sitting on the floor and pulling your toes back toward you and holding this position for an extended period of time. It also helps to stretch out your calf muscles before you go to bed and certainly before you play (see Chapters Five and Six for calf stretches).

Often, the best preventive measure you can take against plantar fasciitis and other foot and ankle injuries is to get custom-made orthotics. According to Dr. Positano, these shock-absorbing inserts remove pressure and stress from painful areas in the foot and ankle, and also promote the proper alignment of the feet. They can restore balance, improve sports performance, and even alleviate pain in the knee, hip, and lower back.

People with flat feet (pes planus) or high arches (cavus foot) are very likely to develop foot and ankle problems if they don't get fitted for orthotics, says Positano. "These foot types can wreak havoc, especially on runners and golfers who stand and walk on their feet as much as they do," he says.

CHAPTER EIGHTEEN

RESUMING ACTIVITY AFTER INJURY

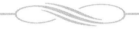

A CASE STUDY: L4-5 FACET PAIN

Bill, a fifty-two-year-old businessman from New York, flies to Los Angeles one March morning for his monthly sales meeting. Unlike his two previous trips to California, however, Bill plans to play eighteen holes of golf the next morning before flying back east. It will be his first round of golf since November, and his first opportunity to test the new 460cc driver his wife bought him for Christmas.

Bill and several colleagues arrive twenty minutes prior to their 7:30 A.M. tee time. Bill fights off some early rustiness to post three consecutive pars on holes four through six. He then unleashes a monstrous drive on the 7th hole, but it comes with a price. Bill finishes awkwardly and feels a twinge of pain in his lower back. He pushes through the pain for the next few holes, but by the time he reaches the 10th tee the pain is radiating into his buttocks and he's having difficulty walking and making a swing. His first round of the new season is cut short after just nine holes, and an uncomfortable five-hour flight awaits him in a few hours' time.

What happened to Bill is not unusual among frequent business travelers. Combine the air-time with the long layoff he's had from golf, and he's a prime candidate for an L4-5 facet-joint injury to his lower back. The facet joints are responsible for rotating the spine, bending it forward, and extending it backward—three movements that occur in every golf swing. As mentioned in Chapter Fifteen, the pressurized cabin in airplanes puts tremendous pressure on the joints and disks in the lower back, leaving business fliers very susceptible to such an injury. In Bill's case, the flying was just part of the problem. A four-month layoff from golf left his core muscles fatigued and in no condition to absorb some of the shock (forces) placed on the facet joints by so many swings.

With this type of injury, Bill won't be seeing the golf course again for quite some time. But if he follows the four-phase program outlined below, he can expect to be back on the course again by May, leaving ample time to enjoy a long, productive season.

The four phases of recovery that follow are designed to return someone with L4-5 facet pain to full golf activity in eight weeks, provided the injury is acute and doesn't require surgery. As with any acute injury, you should see a doctor if the pain hasn't subsided within seven days of suffering the injury.

WEEK 1

Phase 1: Modified Rest

- No exercise for the first three days.
- Ice your lower back for fifteen minutes three times a day. Lie on your back with your legs bent and feet propped up on a chair as you apply the ice.
- Take 800 mg of ibuprofen twice a day (four Advil tablets) with food for three days if not contraindicated.
- On day four, switch to heat in the morning (for fifteen minutes) and ice at night. Continue for the next three days.

- Take two capsules of Zingerflex (www.zingerflex.com) twice daily along with your normal dosage of ibuprofen. Zingerflex is a joint-health supplement that combines ginger, glucosamine, and chondroitin to help reduce inflammation in the joints.

WEEKS 2-3

Phase 2: Golf-Specific Early Rehabilitation

- Perform the exercises in *Back Rx* Series A three times a week to restore general flexibility to your lower back and condition your spine to tolerate more stress. Make sure to get clearance from your doctor before resuming any exercise program after injury.

    (NOTE: *Golf Rx* should not be performed if you're actively suffering from back pain. Resume the exercises in *Golf Rx* when full range of motion returns to the injured area.)
- Take two capsules of Zingerflex twice daily with food.
- Ride a stationary bike (preferably with back support) for twenty minutes, a minimum of three times a week.
- Apply heat to your back in the morning and ice at night (fifteen minutes each), just before you go to bed.

WEEKS 4-5

Phase 3: Golf-Specific Late Rehabilitation
with Partial Return to Sports

- Continue to do the exercises in *Back Rx* Series A three times a week.
- Resume putting, chipping, and pitching. Hit partial wedge shots only; don't exceed a half swing.

- Continue to ride a stationary bike a minimum of three times a week.
- Apply heat to your back in the morning and ice at night.

WEEKS 6-7

Phase 4: Partial Return to Sports

- Resume playing golf, but no more than nine holes, no more than twice a week. Swing at 60 to 70 percent of your normal tempo, no more. Now is not the time to be reaching back for a few extra yards.
- Continue taking Zingerflex and applying heat and ice to your back.
- Continue to ride a bike, walk, or train on an elliptical machine three times a week (twenty minutes per session) for aerobic fitness; resume the exercises in *Back Rx* Series A three times per week.

WEEK 8

Phase 5: Full Return to Golf

- Do not resume golf, even putting, until full range of motion returns to the area affected by the injury. You should be able to bend fully forward (flexion) and backward (extension) without experiencing any pain.
- If you're flying and plan to play golf the next day, make sure to ice your back for fifteen to twenty minutes as soon as you arrive at your hotel. It also helps to take an anti-inflammatory such as Advil (400 to 600 mg if not contraindicated) an hour prior to teeing off, especially if you have a history of lower-back pain.
- Consider an anti-inflammatory diet regimen if you have arthritis of the facet joint of the spine or other joints along with the Zingerflex supplement. (My previous book, *Arthritis Rx*, details an anti-inflammatory diet plan. See www.arthritisrx.net.)

- See a doctor before you start an exercise program like *Golf Rx*. You should be pain- and symptom-free when beginning the program. Continue with *Golf Rx* during the entire off-season in order to maintain peak golf fitness, and for general conditioning purposes. Combine *Golf Rx* (three times a week) with aerobic exercises such as biking, walking, and elliptical training (three times a week for twenty minutes) and you'll be in excellent shape for the start of the new season.

EPILOGUE
THE FUTURE OF GOLF FITNESS

Professional golf was the last major sport to join the fitness craze, which is hard to believe considering that almost every PGA Tour player today has his own golf-conditioning coach. You're just as likely to see Tiger Woods working out in the fitness trailer prior to a tournament round as you are to find him on the driving range. And it doesn't stop with the professional golfer. Recreational golfers are hitting the gym more often, too, looking for that extra edge that will give them another ten or twenty yards off the tee.

The last five years have seen an explosion of golf-specific fitness routines, videos, and training aids, which is only expected to increase in the coming years. And in terms of sport-specific training, golf figures to be among the most proactive in terms of new research and development in the next several years. In fact, as a follow-up to my original study on hip range-of-motion deficits (which is where the idea of *Golf Rx* originated), I plan to work with the PGA Tour again in 2007 to look at the role hip muscles play in generating and sustaining power in the swing. Of particular interest are the posterior fibers of the gluteus medius, the middle of the three gluteal muscles. While not as large or powerful as the gluteus maximus, the gluteus medius is largely responsible for generating clubhead speed in the golf swing. It is my hypothesis that those golfers who exhibit more strength and endurance in the posterior fibers of the gluteus medius hit the ball farther on average than those who have rapidly fatiguing fibers in this muscle group.

In addition to this study, there have been discussions with Stryker Physiotherapy Associates—the health-care provider for both the PGA Tour and Champions Tour—about bringing a golf-fitness facility to midtown Manhattan sometime in 2007. The facility, which would be called Golf Rx/Strengthen Your Game, would bring to the general public what is available only to PGA Tour players right now—a customized fitness/golf-biomechanics program with access to some of the best sports conditioning coaches and swing instructors in the game. On the fitness side, much of the emphasis will be on endurance (the ability of the muscle to generate power over and over) and negative training (the eccentric, or lowering, phase of an exercise movement). Both of these training methods will play a big role in golf-specific training in the future.

Golf Rx will be influential, too. The exercises, tips, and injury-prevention measures offered in this book will not only enhance your performance on the course, but keep you healthy so you can enjoy the game for years to come. It's the perfect off-season conditioning program for golfers, and a valuable resource on preventive care that you will want to refer to again and again in the years to come.

ACKNOWLEDGMENTS

We would like to thank Bob Donatelli, Ph.D., a physical therapist for the PGA Tour and Director of Golf Rehabilitation at Physiotherapy Associates, for his help with designing the *Golf Rx* program; Patricia Ladis, P.T., for helping us with the sequencing of the program and for her Patricia-isms; and Brian Crowell, Head Golf Professional at GlenArbor Golf Club in Bedford Hills, New York, for helping us better understand the biomechanics of the golf swing. We would also like to thank William Cahill and Kelly Kline for their photography skills.

At Gotham Books we are very fortunate to have a great team of publishers; special thanks to Hilary Terrell for a fantastic job with editing, Ray Lundgren and Sabrina Bowers for their outstanding artwork and design, and William Shinker for believing in and supporting the vision of the *Rx* trilogy.

APPENDIX

RESOURCES ON THE WEB

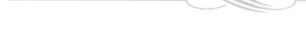

Golf Rx: www.golfrx.org

Official site of the PGA Tour: www.pgatour.com

United States Golf Association: www.usga.org

Stryker Physiotherapy Associates (preferred health-care provider of the PGA Tour
and Champions Tour): www.strengthenyourgame.com

Sports Medicine and Shoulder Service/Hospital for Special Surgery:
www.hss.edu

INDEX